Contemporary Research on Sex Work

Contemporary Research on Sex Work has been co-published simultaneously as *Journal of Psychology & Human Sexuality*, Volume 17, Numbers 1/2 2005.

Monographic Separates from the *Journal of Psychology & Human Sexuality*

For additional information on these and other Haworth Press titles, including descriptions, tables of contents, reviews, and prices, use the QuickSearch catalog at http://www.HaworthPress.com.

Contemporary Research on Sex Work, edited by Jeffrey T. Parsons, PhD (Vol. 17, No. 1/2, 2005). *"This book is a departure from the usual published research in that it takes recent research reports and presents the findings in a straightforward manner. . . . The research it presents is, for the most part, a promising beginning for more collaborative efforts between research and sex workers, which ultimately might lead to intelligent harm reduction programs and legislation based on reality and not morality." (Norma Jean Almodovar, President and Founder, International Sex Worker Foundation for Art, Culture, and Education)*

Adolescence, Sexuality, and the Criminal Law: Multidisciplinary Perspectives, edited by Helmut Graupner, JD, and Vern L. Bullough, PhD (Vol. 16, No. 2/3, 2004). *"There is a great deal of interesting information that one can get from this publication." (Rudolf Müller, Judge, Austrian Supreme Administrative Court; Judge, Austrian Constitutional Court; Honorary Professor of Social Security Law and Labor Law, University of Salzburg)*

Lesbian and Bisexual Women's Mental Health, edited by Robin M. Mathy, MSW, LGSW, MSc, MSt, MA, and Shelly K. Kerr, PhD (Vol. 15, No. 2/3/4, 2003). *Explores the interrelationship between lesbian and bisexual women's mental health and the diverse social contexts in which they live.*

Masturbation as a Means of Achieving Sexual Health, edited by Walter O. Bockting, PhD, and Eli Coleman, PhD (Vol. 14, No. 2/3, 2002). *"Finally, here is an excellent book filled with research illustrating how positive attitudes toward masturbation in history, across cultures, and throughout the life span can help in the achievement of sexual health. This book is an invaluable resource and I highly recommend it for all who are teaching health or sexuality education or are involved in sex counseling and therapy." (William R. Strayton, PhD, ThD, Professor and Coordinator, Human Sexuality Program, Widener University)*

Sex Offender Treatment: Accomplishments, Challenges, and Future Directions, edited by Michael H. Miner, PhD, and Eli Coleman, PhD (Vol. 13, No. 3/4, 2001). *An easy-to-read collection that reviews the major issues and findings on the past decade of research on and treatment of sex offenders. The busy professional will find this book a quick and helpful update for their practice. The reviews presented are succinct, but capture the main issues to be addressed by anyone working with sex offenders." (R. Langevin, PhD, CPsych, Director, Juniper Psychological Services and Associate Professor of Psychiatry, University of Toronto)*

Childhood Sexuality: Normal Sexual Behavior and Development, edited by Theo G. M. Sandfort, PhD, and Jany Rademakers, PhD (Vol. 12, No. 1/2, 2000). *"Important . . . Gives voice to children about their own 'normal' sexual curiosities and desires, and about their behavior and development." (Gunter Schmidt, PhD, Professor, Department of Sex Research, University of Hamburg, Germany)*

Sexual Offender Treatment: Biopsychosocial Perspectives, edited by Eli Coleman, PhD, and Michael Miner, PhD (Vol. 10, No. 3, 2000). *"This guide delivers a diverse look at the complex and intriguing topic of normal child sexuality and the progress that is being made in this area of research."*

New International Directions in HIV Prevention for Gay and Bisexual Men, edited by Michael T. Wright, LICSW, B. R. Simon Rosser, PhD, MPH, and Onno de Zwart, MA (Vol. 10, No. 3/4, 1998). *"Performs a great service to HIV prevention research and health promotion. . . . It takes the words of gay and bisexual men seriously by locating men's sexual practice in their love relationships and casual sex encounters and examines their responses to HIV." (Susan Kippax, Associate Professor and Director, National Center in HIV Social Research, School of Behavioral Sciences, Macquarie University, New South Wales, Australia)*

Jeffrey T. Parsons, PhD
Editor

Contemporary Research
on Sex Work

Cor   ıed
sim   *lity,*

Volume 17, Numbers 1/2 2005.

Pre-publication
REVIEWS,
COMMENTARIES,
EVALUATIONS . . .

"This book updates and expands the literature on sexual oppression and its effects. From prostitution to HIV/AIDS, readers will have a very handy compilation of a variety of methods for analyzing and understanding some very complicated issues."

Dr. Joel Fischer, ACSW
Professor, University of Hawai'i
School of Social Work, Honolulu

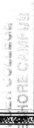

"All too often, academic research on sex work treats the subjects involved–the sex workers–as if we are nothing more than bugs under a microscope, entities without lives, families, hopes, dreams, and jobs. This book is a departure from the usual published research in that it takes recent research reports and presents the findings in a straightforward manner. It does not condemn sex work or sex workers, and it is not presumed that sex workers are incapable of intelligent, rational behavior simply because we engage in commercial sexual activity. The research it presents is, for the most part, a promising beginning for more collaborative efforts between research and sex workers, which ultimately might lead to intelligent harm reduction programs and legislation based on reality and not morality."

Norma Jean Almodovar
President and Founder
International Sex Worker Foundation
for Art, Culture, and Education

The Haworth Press, Inc.

Sexuality Education in Postsecondary and Professional Training Settings, edited by James W. Maddock (Vol. 9, No. 3/4, 1997). *"A diverse group of contributers all experienced sexuality educators–offer summary information, critical commentary, thoughtful analysis, and projections of future trends in sexuality education in postsecondary settings. . . . The chapters present valuable resources, ranging from historical references to contemporary Websites."* (Adolescence)

Sexual Coercion in Dating Relationships, edited by E. Sandra Byers and Lucia F. O'Sullivan (Vol. 8, No. 1/2, 1996). *"Tackles a big issue with the best tools presently available to social and health scientists. . . . Perhaps the most remarkable thing about these excellent chapters is the thread of optimism that remains despite the depressing topic. Each author . . . chips away at oppression and acknowledges the strength of women who have experienced sexual coercion while struggling to eliminate sexist assumptions that deny women sexual autonomy and pleasure."* (Naomi B. McCormick, PhD, Professor, Department of Psychology, State University of New York at Plattsburgh)

HIV/AIDS and Sexuality, edited by Michael W. Ross (Vol. 7, No. 1/2, 1995). *"An entire volume on the topic of HIV and sexuality, bringing together a number of essays and studies, which cover a wide range of relevant issues. It really is a relief to finally read some research and thoughts about sexual functioning and satisfaction in HIV-positive persons."* (Association of Lesbian and Gay Psychologists)

Gender Dysphoria: Interdisciplinary Approaches in Clinical Management, edited by Walter O. Bockting and Eli Coleman (Vol. 5, No. 4, 1993). *"A useful modern summary of the state-of--the-art endocrine and psychiatric approach to this important problem."* (Stephen B. Levine, MD, Clinical Professor of Psychiatry, School of Medicine, Case Western Reserve University; Co-Director, Center for Marital and Sexual Health)

Sexual Transmission of HIV Infection: Risk Reduction, Trauma, and Adaptation, edited by Lena Nilsson Schönnesson, PhD (Vol. 5, No. 1/2, 1992). *"This is an essential title for understanding how AIDS and HIV are perceived and treated in modern America."* (The Bookwatch)

John Money: A Tribute, edited by Eli Coleman (Vol. 4, No. 2, 1991). *"Original, provocative, and breaks new ground."* (Science Books & Films)

Contemporary Research on Sex Work

Jeffrey T. Parsons, PhD
Editor

Contemporary Research on Sex Work has been co-published simultaneously as *Journal of Psychology & Human Sexuality*, Volume 17, Numbers 1/2 2005.

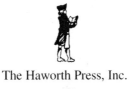

The Haworth Press, Inc.

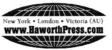

New York • London • Victoria (AU)
www.HaworthPress.com

Contemporary Research on Sex Work has been co-published simultaneously as *Journal of Psychology & Human Sexuality*™, Volume 17, Numbers 1/2 2005.

Cover design by Kerry E. Mack

The Haworth Press, Inc., 10 Alice Street, Binghamton, NY 13904-1580 USA

Library of Congress Cataloging-in-Publication Data

Contemporary research on sex work / Jeffrey T. Parsons, editor.
    p. ơm.
    "Co-published simultaneously as Journal of psychology & human sexuality, volume 17, numbers 1/2 2005."
    Includes bibliographical references and index.
    ISBN-13: 978-0-7890-2963-8 (hc. : alk. paper)
    ISBN-10: 0-7890-2963-4 (hc. : alk. paper)
    ISBN-13: 978-0-7890-2964-5 (pbk. : alk. paper)
    ISBN-10: 0-7890-2964-2 (pbk. : alk. paper)
    1. Prostitution–Research. 2. Prostitutes–Social conditions. 3. Prostitutes–Health and hygiene.
    4. Hygiene, Sexual. I. Parsons, Jeffrey T. II. Journal of psychology & human sexuality.
HQ118.C66 2005
306.74–dc22
                                                                        2005002156

Indexing, Abstracting & Website/Internet Coverage

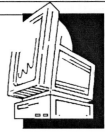

This section provides you with a list of major indexing & abstracting services and other tools for bibliographic access. That is to say, each service began covering this periodical during the year noted in the right column. Most Websites which are listed below have indicated that they will either post, disseminate, compile, archive, cite or alert their own Website users with research-based content from this work. (This list is as current as the copyright date of this publication.)

Abstracting, Website/Indexing Coverage . . . . Year When Coverage Began

- *Business Source Corporate: coverage of nearly 3,350 quality magazines and journals; designed to meet the diverse information needs of corporations; EBSCO Publishing <http://www.epnet.com/corporate/bsourcecorp.asp>* 2001

- *Cambridge Scientific Abstracts is a leading publisher of scientific information in print journals, online databases, CD-ROM and via the Internet <http://www.csa.com>* 1992

- *EBSCOhost Electronic Journals Service (EJS) <http://ejournals.ebsco.com>* 2002

- *Educational Administration Abstracts (EAA)* 1995

- *e-psyche, LLC <http://www.e-psyche.net>* 2001

- *Family & Society Studies Worldwide <http://www.nisc.com>* 1996

- *Family Index Database <http://www.familyscholar.com>* 2003

- *Family Violence & Sexual Assault Bulletin.* 1991

- *GenderWatch <http://www.slinfo.com>* 1999

- *Google <http://www.google.com>* 2004

- *Google Scholar <http://www.scholar.google.com>.* 2004

- *Haworth Document Delivery Center <http://www.HaworthPress.com/journals/dds.asp>* 1988

(continued)

*Exact start date to come.

*Special Bibliographic Notes related to special journal issues
(separates) and indexing/abstracting:*

- indexing/abstracting services in this list will also cover material in any "separate" that is co-published simultaneously with Haworth's special thematic journal issue or DocuSerial. Indexing/abstracting usually covers material at the article/chapter level.
- monographic co-editions are intended for either non-subscribers or libraries which intend to purchase a second copy for their circulating collections.
- monographic co-editions are reported to all jobbers/wholesalers/approval plans. The source journal is listed as the "series" to assist the prevention of duplicate purchasing in the same manner utilized for books-in-series.
- to facilitate user/access services all indexing/abstracting services are encouraged to utilize the co-indexing entry note indicated at the bottom of the first page of each article/chapter/contribution.
- this is intended to assist a library user of any reference tool (whether print, electronic, online, or CD-ROM) to locate the monographic version if the library has purchased this version but not a subscription to the source journal.
- individual articles/chapters in any Haworth publication are also available through the Haworth Document Delivery Service (HDDS).

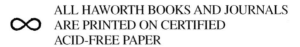

Contemporary Research on Sex Work

CONTENTS

ABOUT THE EDITOR

Jeffrey T. Parsons, PhD, is Professor of Psychology at Hunter College and the Graduate Center of the City University of New York (CUNY), and is also the Director of Hunter's Center for HIV/AIDS Educational Studies and Training (CHEST). His research has focused on HIV prevention efforts, particularly among gay and bisexual men and those living with HIV, as well as sexual health issues, and has been funded by the Centers for Disease Control and Prevention, National Institute on Alcohol Abuse and Alcoholism, and National Institute on Drug Abuse. In addition, Dr. Parsons has conducted research in the areas of sex work, sexual compulsivity, and substance use/abuse. He is currently the President-Elect of the Society for the Scientific Study of Sexuality (SSSS), the Vice President of the Society for the Advancement of Sexual Health (SASH), and a member of the Committee on Psychology and AIDS (COPA) of the American Psychological Association.

Researching the World's Oldest Profession: Introduction

Jeffrey T. Parsons, PhD

This volume presents eleven papers which represent contemporary research into the world of commercial sex. Social scientists from a number of disciplines, including psychology, sociology, and public health, have explored varied facets of sex work. Diversity is the emphasis of this volume. Diverse methodological approaches, including targeted sampling, qualitative and quantitative interviews, ethnographic interviews with key informants, using sex workers as recruiters, and quasi-experimental intervention designs are featured.

For many years, the focus of sex work research was on street-based male and female sex workers, and recently many investigations have focused on HIV-related risks, typically in terms of the risks that sex workers pose to their clients. Certainly, some of the papers in this publication continue to try and better understand HIV risk among street-based sex workers. However, there is also a focus on other types of sex workers, such as escorts, call girls, and those who work in massage parlors, bars/nightclubs, cantinas, and brothels. Further, although many of the articles do emphasize sexual risk practices related to HIV, most of the

Jeffrey T. Parsons is affiliated with the Graduate Center of the City University of New York, the Center for HIV/AIDS Educational Studies and Training (CHEST), and Hunter College of the City University of New York.

Address correspondence to: Jeffrey T. Parsons, Professor, Department of Psychology, Hunter College of the City University of New York, 695 Park Avenue, New York, NY 10021 (E-mail: jeffrey.parsons@hunter.cuny.edu).

[Haworth co-indexing entry note]: "Researching the World's Oldest Profession: Introduction." Parsons, Jeffrey T. Co-published simultaneously in *Journal of Psychology & Human Sexuality* (The Haworth Press, Inc.) Vol. 17, No. 1/2, 2005, pp. 1-3; and: *Contemporary Research on Sex Work* (ed: Jeffrey T. Parsons) The Haworth Press, Inc., 2005, pp. 1-3. Single or multiple copies of this article are available for a fee from The Haworth Document Delivery Service [1-800-HAWORTH, 9:00 a.m. - 5:00 p.m. (EST). E-mail address: docdelivery@haworthpress.com].

articles move beyond a basic association between sex work and unprotected sex, in order to better contextualize sexual risk, and to more fully describe the lives of those in the sex industry. The research presented comes from the United States (Los Angeles, Miami, New York City), Cambodia, Philippines, Argentina, and Canada, and includes sex workers that are male, female, and transgendered.

The diverse set of papers in this volume provides a number of important insights into research on sex workers, particularly dispelling any notions that sex workers represent a homogenous group. Several key points are discussed in the papers. First, venue matters. Those who work more independently are different from those who work on the streets. Second, gender matters. Female sex workers often face different barriers and issues to their work than males. Third, policy matters. The different ways that various countries and communities attempt to criminalize or regulate sex work have a clear impact on the lives of sex workers. Fourth, and finally, all three of these factors: venue, gender, and policy, have clear and direct effects on power and control in sex work interactions. This can, in turn, have a direct impact on health, social functioning, mental health, and HIV/STI risks.

There is a clear need for high quality research of sex workers and their clients in order to either confirm or dispel stereotypes, often resulting from research studies with problematic methodologies or single studies on a very narrowly defined population. Further, the time has come to begin to take our understanding of sex work and begin to explore interventions and programs designed to improve the social and physical lives of sex workers and their clients. The papers included in this volume make an effort to begin this process.

Reback and her colleagues present their work with transgendered female sex workers in Los Angeles, and find, contrary to expectations, that those women who engaged in sex work were more likely to use condoms than those that did not engage in sex work. Busza describes preliminary work in Cambodia in which sex workers themselves were engaged in the participatory process leading to the development of an intervention. A behavioral intervention, led by Morisky and colleagues, was directed at the individual sex worker level, as well as the organizational level in the Philippines, and was successful in increasing condom use. Another study, led by Surratt and her colleagues, presents baseline data from a larger intervention trial for street-based female sex workers in Miami. Koken and her colleagues examine sex workers and clients, and those who report both being paid for and paying for sex among men in the gay community of New York City. Morrison and Whitehead examine stigma resistance among male sex workers in Canada, and Disogra and his colleagues examine the use and barriers to the use of health services among male sex workers in Argentina. Abramovich provides a in-depth analysis of the previous literature on childhood sexual abuse and sex work.

Some papers, through the use of qualitative methods, go beyond previous research findings to actually provide some understanding and context for those findings. For example, previous studies have documented that some sex workers are more likely to use condoms with paying partners rather than with partners in their private lives. Jackson and her colleagues delve deeply into the relational issues to identify potential reasons for this finding among female sex workers in Canada. Lever and colleagues utilize ethnographic interviews with a wide range of sex workers, and informed others (e.g., police officers, owners and managers of sex work establishments), to better understand the intersection between race/ethnicity and venue and how this affects the lives of female sex workers in Los Angeles. Lewis and her colleagues explore female, male, and transgendered sex workers in Canada, specifically focusing on issues of job-related risk and safety, and how these are driven by the legal and policy contexts.

Overall, the papers help to take us into the next generation of sex work research, highlighting the need to understand sex work as work, rather than making assumptions of pathology among those in the sex industry. Clearly, there are those sex workers who face a myriad of problems and challenges, such as HIV, drug abuse, violence, and a lack of power and control over their lives. However, this commonly held view of sex workers fails to fully capture the diversity of those in the sex industry, and further research and intervention efforts must continue to carefully consider the impact of venue, gender, and policy on the lives of sex workers and their clients, as well as to explore varied methodologies in order to more comprehensively understand the world of sex work.

ACKNOWLEDGMENTS

This volume owes much to many. First, I would like to thank Eli Coleman and Annie Picken for their support and assistance with the production of this collection. Second, I would like to thank Diane Tider for her valuable assistance in organizing and coordinating the submission, review, and acceptance process. Third, I would like to thank David Bimbi and Juline Koken, the two doctoral students who have had a tremendous influence on my interest in and approach to the study of sex work. Finally, I would like to thank the many reviewers who participated in the process.

HIV Seroprevalence and Risk Behaviors Among Transgendered Women Who Exchange Sex in Comparison with Those Who Do Not

Cathy J. Reback, PhD
Emilia L. Lombardi, PhD
Paul A. Simon, MD, MPH
Douglas M. Frye, MD, MPH

Cathy J. Reback is affiliated with the Van Ness Recovery House, Friends Research Institute, Inc., and the Integrated Substance Abuse Programs (ISAP), UCLA, Los Angeles, CA.

Emilia L. Lombardi is affiliated with the Department of Infectious Diseases/Microbiology, University of Pittsburgh, Pittsburgh, PA.

Paul A. Simon and Douglas M. Frye are affiliated with the Los Angeles County Department of Health Services, Los Angeles, California.

Address correspondence to: Cathy J. Reback, PhD, Van Ness Recovery House, Friends Research Institute, Inc., 1136 N. La Brea Avenue, West Hollywood, CA 90038 (E-mail: Rebackcj@aol.com).

The authors would like to thank the following persons and organizations for their help and participation in this study: Cathleen Bemis, MS, Bobby Gatson, Sharon Lu, MPH, Gordon Bunch, MA, the study interviewers, Asian Pacific AIDS Intervention Team, Van Ness Recovery House, Bienestar, Minority AIDS Project, and the Los Angeles transgendered women's communities.

This study was generously supported by the University of California Universitywide AIDS Research Program grant #PC97-LAC-012L and the California State Office of AIDS.

[Haworth co-indexing entry note]: "HIV Seroprevalence and Risk Behaviors Among Transgendered Women Who Exchange Sex in Comparison with Those Who Do Not." Reback, Cathy J. et al. Co-published simultaneously in *Journal of Psychology & Human Sexuality* (The Haworth Press, Inc.) Vol. 17, No. 1/2, 2005, pp. 5-22; and: *Contemporary Research on Sex Work* (ed: Jeffrey T. Parsons) The Haworth Press, Inc., 2005, pp. 5-22. Single or multiple copies of this article are available for a fee from The Haworth Document Delivery Service [1-800-HAWORTH, 9:00 a.m. - 5:00 p.m. (EST). E-mail address: docdelivery@haworthpress.com].

SUMMARY. Many transgendered women face social, cultural, and economic challenges that result in their reliance on exchange sex to secure needed items. This study compares the HIV seroprevalence and risk behaviors of transgendered women who exchanged sex with those who did not. Of the 244 transgendered women interviewed, those who exchanged sex comprised 58.2% of the sample and were younger (p < .001), less educated (p < .001), and less likely to have or seek health care (p < .001). HIV seroprevalence was higher in those who exchanged sex than those who did not (26.1% versus 16.7%). Those who exchanged sex reported more casual sex partners and were more likely to report sex while high on alcohol and/or drugs, but were also more likely to report condom use. In the multivariate analysis, exchange sex was not associated with increased HIV seroprevalance, but substance use during sex and African-American race were associated with increased seroprevalance. These findings highlight the importance of examining the sexual lives and social circumstances of transgendered women and the necessity of integrating substance abuse treatment into HIV prevention settings. *[Article copies available for a fee from The Haworth Document Delivery Service: 1-800-HAWORTH. E-mail address: <docdelivery@haworthpress.com> Website: <http://www.HaworthPress.com> © 2005 by The Haworth Press, Inc. All rights reserved.]*

KEYWORDS. Transgender, HIV seroprevalence, risk behavior, exchange sex

Many transgendered women (i.e., male-to-female transgendered individuals) are at risk for high unemployment, low income, lower levels of education, and unstable housing (Nemoto et al., 1999; Reback, Simon, Bemis & Gatson, 2001). Economic necessity, as a result of severe unemployment and housing discrimination (Lombardi, Wilchins, Priesing & Malouf, 2001; Sykes, 1999), often results in a reliance on exchange sex to secure money, drugs, shelter, food and other needed items (Kammerer, Mason, Connors & Durkee, 2001).

Although transgendered women are generally perceived to be at increased risk for HIV infection, there is relatively little objective HIV risk information available on this population (Bockting, Robinson & Rosser, 1998; Bockting, Rosser & Scheltema, 1999; Boehmer, 2002). While some studies have assessed HIV seroprevalence and risk behaviors among transgendered women in general (Clements-Nolle, Marx,

Guzman & Katz, 2001; Kenagy, 2002; Nemoto et al., 1999; Stephens, Cozza & Braithwaite, 1999), most published reports have focused specifically on transgendered women who engage in sex work (Belza et al., 2000; Boles & Elifson, 1994; Harcourt et al., 2001; Spizzichino et al., 2001; Weinberg, Shaver & Williams, 1999) and a few studies compared HIV risks of transgendered women who exchange sex with non-transgendered individuals who exchange sex (Elifson et al., 1993; Gras et al., 1997; Inciardi & Surratt, 1997; Modan et al., 1992; Verster et al., 2001). These studies, which are geographically unique (Atlanta, Georgia, USA; Amsterdam, the Netherlands; Rio de Janeiro, Brazil; Tel Aviv, Israel; and Rome, Italy), all found that transgendered women sex workers have a greater HIV seroprevalence than their non-transgendered counterparts. In these studies, their high HIV rates have been associated with substance use and receptive anal sex without condom use. Only one has compared the HIV risk behaviors of women involved in sex work with those that were not (Reback & Lombardi, 2001) and found that sex work was associated with greater substance use and a greater number of non-exchange male sexual partners. However, this study also demonstrated that HIV risk was lower among sex workers due to their higher use of condoms.

Two studies in San Francisco compared risk factors of transgendered women with gay and bisexual males and heterosexual females (Nemoto et al., 1999; Weinberg, Shaver & Williams, 1999). Transgendered women had more non-exchange sexual partners (Weinberg, Shaver & Williams, 1999) and had more exchange partners and engaged in more risky sexual behaviors when conducting sex work than a comparison group of gay and bisexual male and female sex workers (Nemoto et al., 1999).

Recent studies indicate that many transgendered women continue to be at high risk for HIV. At a San Francisco counseling and testing site, an HIV seroconversion rate of 7.8 per 100 person-years was found in transgendered women (Kellogg et al., 2001). In Los Angeles, there were 3.4 incident infections per 100 person-years among participants in a local transgender health study (Simon, Reback & Bemis, 2000). Additionally, an incidence of 5.6 per 100 person-years was found among transgendered women who received repeat HIV testing at public counseling and testing sites in Los Angeles–higher than for any other demographic group (Croker, personal communication, December 2003).

Based on the current literature, it is unclear the degree to which HIV risk and patterns of risk behavior differ among transgendered women who exchange sex from those who do not. This paper reports on the results of a study that examined HIV seroprevalence and sexual and drug-using risk behaviors among transgendered women who did and did not exchange sex and were receiving HIV prevention services in Los Angeles, California. We predict that there are important differences in the HIV risk profiles of transgendered women who exchange sex versus those who do not. The objective of this study was to assess whether or not these predicted differences exist and, if so, to characterize these differences and, thereby, better inform HIV prevention interventions targeted to transgendered women.

METHODS

Participants and Procedures

The Los Angeles Transgender Health Study was a research and community collaboration designed for the collection of epidemiological and behavioral data on transgendered women. To be eligible for participation in the study, persons had to be at least 18 years of age, reside in Los Angeles County, and identify themselves as either transgender, transsexual, or a woman born as a male. Males who dressed as women but identified as men (e.g., crossdressers) were excluded from the study, as were transgendered men (female-to-male transgendered individuals).

Participants were recruited between February 1998 and January 1999 from three community agencies and in outreach settings where HIV prevention services were being delivered. These services ranged from brief one-time encounters to structured interventions involving multiple contacts. The agencies are located in the urban center of the county, but operate in different neighborhoods. One agency serves predominantly Latinos, another predominantly Asians, and the last serves a racially mixed clientele. A fourth agency, serving predominantly African-American clientele, was initially included in the study, but subsequently excluded from the analysis due to data collection inconsistencies and irregularities in the data (Reback, Simon, Bemis & Gatson, 2001; Reback & Simon, 2004).

After obtaining informed consent (approved by the Health Research Association Institutional Review Board), participants each received a 30-45 minute face-to-face interview using a standardized questionnaire, which was adapted from the instrument used in a San Francisco study (Clements-Nolle et al., 2001). The questionnaire consisted of seven modules: screening eligibility; demographics and socioeconomic status; health care access and medical history; sexual behavior; alcohol and drug use; psychosocial and legal issues; and HIV prevention. Trained interviewers, all of whom identified as transgendered women, administered the questionnaire in English or Spanish. During the development of the instrument the questionnaire was "back" translated from English to Spanish and back to English to ensure accuracy. Following the interview, participants received an oral fluid-based HIV-1 antibody test from OraSure Technologies. All specimens found to be positive by enzyme immunoassay (EIA) were then confirmed with a Western Blot assay.

A total of 244 transgendered women were enrolled in the study. Participants had a mean age of 30 years (range from 18 to 60 years); 49% were Latina, 21% Asian/Pacific Islander, 15% Caucasian, 7% African American, 2% American Indian, and 6% mixed or other. Sixty-three percent were born outside the United States. Fifty-six percent identified their gender as female or woman, 39% as transgender or transsexual, and 5% as other; 77% identified their sexuality as heterosexual, 7% gay, 6% bisexual, 1% lesbian, and 9% as other. Although 30% reported having had surgery to enhance their gender presentation, only 3% reported genital reconstructive surgery. Participants had completed an average of 11 years of schooling and 50% earned less than $12,000 a year. Sixty-six percent of the participants reported having a regular source of health care; 10% had either no source of care or relied on the emergency room; and 24% reported not having sought health care. Only 36% of participants reported having health insurance.

Data Analysis

Analyses were done to compare HIV seroprevalence and risk behaviors among those who exchanged sex in the previous six months with those who did not. For the purpose of this study, an exchange sexual partner was defined as a sexual partner with whom sex is exchanged for a needed item such as money, drugs, shelter or food. Therefore, in this context, an exchange partner did not refer to someone who exchanged sex for an emotional reward such as love or a sense of security. A main sex partner was defined as someone with whom the participant had a close, intimate relationship; a casual sex partner was someone with whom they had sex, but whom they did not consider to be their main partner.

Demographic variables include age, primary gender identification, sexual identification, race/ethnicity, birth country, years lived in the United States (for those born outside of the United States), education, income, whether they have health insurance, and their source of regular health care. Age was dichotomized in order to focus attention on generational differences. For example, those under 30 years of age may have been exposed to HIV education during their formative sexual years. Income earned in the last 30 days consists of seven categories (less than $50, $51-$249, $250-$499, $500-$999, $1,000-$2,999, $3,000-$4,999, $5,000 or more) that were used as a continuous variable for multivariate analysis but were dichotomized (i.e., earns less than $12,000 a year, earns more than $12,000 a year) for bivariate analyses.

Risk behaviors were assessed, using a six-month recall period, by asking (1) how many main, casual, and exchange partners participants had in the previous six months; (2) whether participants reported receptive or insertive anal intercourse with those partners (separately); (3) how often condoms were used when they had anal intercourse (never or almost never versus higher levels of condom use); (4) whether they injected drugs and, if so, whether they used a needle obtained from the streets to inject drugs; (5) whether they injected hormones and, if so, whether they used a needle obtained from the streets to inject non-prescribed and unmonitored hormones; and (6) whether they had sex while high on alcohol and/or drugs. The study compared those who reported any exchange sexual partners in the previous six months with those who did not report an exchange sexual partner in the previous six months.

Analyses were done using SAS version 8.02. Differences between categorical variables were evaluated for statistical significance with the Chi-square test and differences between continuous variables were assessed with the F-test within proc anova. Fisher exact tests were used in analysis of condom use as small sample sizes made Chi-square unreliable. P-values of < 0.05 were considered statistically significant (p-values of < .10 were also identified but just to note marginal significance). Bivariate comparisons of HIV seroprevalance were assessed by calculating odds ratios (ORs). Multivariate comparisons of seroprevalence were evaluated using logistic regression to calculate adjusted ORs with 95% confidence intervals (CIs). Multiple linear regression was used to analyze continuous variables.

RESULTS

Comparison of Sociodemographic Characteristics by Exchange Sex Status

Table 1 compares the sociodemographic characteristics of those who reported exchange sex versus those who did not. Those who reported

TABLE 1. Comparison of sociodemographic characteristics among transgendered women who exchanged sex in the previous six months and those who did not.

CHARACTERISTIC	Full Sample N = 244		Exchanged Sex n = 142		Did Not Exchange Sex n = 102		P-value[a]
	n (%) or Mean (SD)		n (%) or Mean (SD)		n (%) or Mean (SD)		
Age Group[b] Mean (SD)	29.79	(SD = 8.18)	27.80	(SD = 6.75)	32.57	(SD = 9.17)	<.001
Gender Identity[c]							
Female	136	(56.2)	91	(64.1)	45	(44.1)	<.01
Transgender/transsexual	94	(38.8)	47	(33.1)	47	(46.1)	<.05
Sexual Identity							
Heterosexual	187	(76.6)	127	(89.4)	60	(58.8)	<.001
Heterosexual female identification	122	(50)	86	(60.6)	36	(35.3)	<.001
Race/Ethnicity							
African American	18	(7.4)	7	(4.9)	11	(10.8)	NS
Asian	50	(20.5)	24	(16.9)	26	(25.5)	NS
Caucasian	37	(15.2)	10	(7.0)	27	(26.5)	<.001
Latina	120	(49.2)	91	(64.1)	29	(28.4)	<.001
Other/multiethnic	19	(7.8)	10	(7.04)	9	(8.82)	NS
Country of Birth							
United States	91	(37.3)	36	(25.4)	55	(53.9)	
Other (including US territories)	153	(62.7)	106	(74.7)	47	(46.4)	<.001
Number of years living in US[d] Mean (SD)	8.64	(SD = 5.92)	7.59	(SD = 5.36)	11.00	(SD = 6.50)	<.001
Education[e] Mean (SD)	11.09	(SD = 3.35)	10.24	(SD = 3.43)	12.27	(SD = 2.85)	<.001
Annual income[f]							
Less than $12,000	123	(50.4)	70	(49.3)	53	(52.0)	
$12,000 or more	121	(49.6)	72	(50.7)	49	(48.0)	NS
Surgery to enhance gender presentation							
Any[c]	73	(30.2)	46	(32.9)	27	(26.5)	NS
Breast augmentation	52	(21.3)	36	(25.4)	16	(15.7)	NS
Rhinoplasty	45	(18.4)	34	(23.9)	11	(10.8)	<.01
Genital reconstructive/vaginoplasty	7	(2.9)	1	(0.7)	6	(5.9)	<.05
Health insurance coverage[c]							
Yes	86	(35.5)	25	(17.7)	61	(60.4)	<.001
No	156	(64.5)	116	(82.3)	40	(39.6)	
Regular source of health care							
Has source	162	(66.4)	75	(52.8)	87	(85.3)	<.001
No source or emergency room	24	(9.8)	17	(12.0)	7	(6.9)	NS
Has not sought health care	58	(23.8)	50	(35.2)	8	(7.8)	<.001
HIV Seroprevalence	54	(22.1)	37	(26.1)	17	(16.7)	NS

[a]NS indicates difference was not statistically significant at p < 0.05; [b]Ages ranged from 18 to 60 years; [c]Data does not include two missing cases; [d]Among foreign-born study subjects only; n = 153; [e]Data does not include one missing case; [f]Estimated from reported income in recent month. Mean annual income = $12,000. Data excludes 2 missing cases.

exchange sex were significantly younger (28 versus 33 years of age), less educated (an average of 10 versus 12 years of school), more likely to self-identify as female (64% versus 44%), and less likely to have had genital reconstructive surgery (< 1% versus 6%). A higher percentage of transgendered women who exchanged sex were Latina (64% versus 28%), foreign-born (75% versus 46%) and, among foreign-born, had been in the country for fewer years than those who did not exchange sex (8 years versus 11 years). Those who exchanged sex were less likely to have health insurance (18% versus 60%) or a regular source of health care (53% versus 85%), and were more likely not to have sought health care (35% versus 8%).

Bivariate Analyses of HIV Seroprevalence

HIV test results were obtained on all 244 participants (Table 2), 54 (22%) of whom tested positive and one test was indeterminate. Participants who were 30 years of age and older had two and a half times the odds of being HIV seropositive than did younger participants (OR = 2.70; 95% CI = 1.44, 5.07). Those who made more than the mean income of $12,000 per year were nearly three times less likely to test HIV positive than those with a lower income (OR = .38; 95% CI = .20, .72). Those who completed 12 or more years of schooling were less than half as likely to test positive than those who completed less than 12 years of schooling (OR = .48; 95% CI = .26, .90). African-American participants were three times more likely to test positive than other race/ethnicities (OR = 3.13; 95% CI = 1.17, 8.38) and Asians were least likely to test positive (OR = .11; 95% CI = .03, .48). Lastly, those who engaged in exchange sex were nearly twice as likely to test positive (OR = 1.76; 95% CI = .93, 3.35).

HIV Risk Behaviors Among Those Who Exchanged Sex and Those Who Did Not

Table 3 compares high-risk behaviors of those who reported exchange sex and those who reported sex but did not report exchange sex. Transgendered women who reported exchange sex reported a mean of over 150 exchange partners in the previous six months. Those who reported exchange sex also reported having more casual partners than did those who did not report exchange sex (a mean of 10 versus 2 partners). There was no difference in either group's participation in anal intercourse (both as receptive and/or insertive partners); however, there was

TABLE 2. Comparison of HIV seroprevalence by sociodemographic characteristics.

CHARACTERISTIC			FULL SAMPLE N = 244		
	n	Sero-prevalence	Odds ratio	95% Confidence interval	P-value
Age Group					
30 years or older	112	31.3%	2.70	1.44-5.07	<.01
18-29 years	132	14.4%			
Gender, self-identified					
Female vs all others	136	20.6%	.82	.45-1.50	NS
Transgender/transsexual vs all others	24	26.6%	1.51	.82-2.79	NS
Race/Ethnicity					
African American vs all others	18	44.4%	3.13	1.17-8.38	<.05
Asian vs all others	50	4.0%	.11	.03-.48	<.001
Caucasian vs all others	36	16.2%	.64	.25-1.63	NS
Latina vs all others	120	25.8%	1.53	.83-2.82	NS
Other/multiethnic vs all others	15	40.0%	2.51	.85-7.41	NS
Country of Birth					
United States	91	24.2%	.83	.45-1.54	NS
Other (includes US territories)	153	20.9%			
Education					
Less than 12 years competed	115	28.7%			
12 or more years completed	129	16.3%	.48	.26-.90	<.05
Annual income					
Less than $12,000	123	30.1%			
$12,000 or more	121	14.1%	.38	.20-.72	<.01
Exchange sex status					
Did not exchange sex in previous six months	102	16.7%			
Did exchange sex in previous six months	142	26.1%	1.76	.93-3.35	<.08

a difference in condom use. Transgendered women who did not participate in exchange sex were more likely to report that they never or almost never used a condom during anal intercourse than those who reported exchange sex. Those who engaged in exchange sex were more likely to use condoms during anal intercourse regardless of whether they were the receptive or insertive partner, although unprotected receptive intercourse with a main partner was still high (40%). In both groups, transgendered women were more likely to be the insertive partner during anal intercourse with partners with whom they were not emotionally close (i.e., exchange or casual partners rather than main partners).

TABLE 3. Comparison of selected high-risk behaviors between those who exchanged sex and those who did not.

RISK BEHAVIOR	Exchanged Sex	Did Not Exchange Sex (excludes those who did not report any sex)	P-value[b]
	n = 142	n = 76	
	n (%) or Mean (SD)	n (%) or Mean (SD)	
Number of main partners, Mean (SD)	1.35 (SD = .95)	1.10 (SD = .31)	<.10
Number of casual partners, Mean (SD)	10.27 (SD = 26.76)	1.96 (SD = 3.22)	<.01
Number of exchange partners, Mean (SD)	156.59 (SD = 227.57)	---	
Receptive anal intercourse w/main partner	65 (94.2)	40 (87.0)	<.05
Receptive anal intercourse w/casual partner	91 (90.1)	32 (71.1)	<.01
Receptive anal intercourse w/exchange partner	118 (83.7)		
unprotected anal receptive sex w/main partner[c]	26 (40.0)	20 (50.0)	NS
unprotected anal receptive sex w/casual partner[c]	11 (12.1)	10 (31.3)	<.05
unprotected anal receptive sex w/exchange partner[c]	4 (3.39)		
Insertive anal intercourse w/main partner	8 (11.6)	9 (19.2)	NS
Insertive anal intercourse w/casual partner	27 (27.0)	13 (28.26)	NS
Insertive anal intercourse w/exchange partner	77 (55.0)		
unprotected anal insertive sex w/main partner[d]	2 (25.0)	7 (77.8)	<.10
unprotected anal insertive sex w/casual partner[d]	2 (7.41)	4 (30.8)	<.10
unprotected anal insertive sex w/exchange partner[d]	4 (5.19)		

RISK BEHAVIOR	Exchanged Sex	Did Not Exchange Sex (includes those who did not report any sex)	P-value
	n = 142	n = 102	
	n (%)	n (%)	
Ever injected hormones	107 (75.4)	61 (59.8)	<.01
street needle used for hormones[e]	60 (42.3)	33 (32.4)	NS
Injected drug to get high or buzzed	14 (51.9)	6 (35.3)	NS
shared needle to inject drug[f]	7 (50.0)	1 (16.7)	NS
Had sex while high on alcohol or drug	98 (69.0)	31 (30.4)	<.0001

[a] Those who did not have any type of sex in the previous six months were excluded from the analyses of sexual risk, as were the few that had sex reassignment surgery, but were included in the analysis of injection risks; [b] NS indicates difference was not statistically significant at p < 0.05; [c] Among only those having had anal receptive intercourse, reported intercourse with a condom never or almost never in previous six months; [d] Among only those having had anal insertive intercourse, reported intercourse with a condom never or almost never in previous six months; [e] Among only those using a needle for hormone injection, needle was obtained from non-health care system source. [f] Among only those injecting a drug to get high or buzzed.

Those who exchanged sex were more likely than those who did not exchange sex to report risks with needles and substance use. These transgendered women were more likely to report ever injecting hormones and using needles obtained from street sources. While both groups reported similar experiences with injection drug use, a higher percentage of those who exchanged sex reported sharing their needles (although this difference was not statistically significant). The biggest difference between the two groups was whether they used alcohol and/or drugs during sex. Those who exchanged sex were more likely to report having used alcohol and/or drugs during sex (69%) than those who did not exchange sex (30%).

Multivariate Analyses of HIV Seroprevalence

Table 4 shows differences between the groups in a number of HIV risk behaviors while controlling for ethnicity (Latino versus all other) and education. Those who exchanged sex in the previous six months reported a greater a number of casual sexual partners and were more likely to report receptive anal intercourse. Those who exchanged sex were three and half times more likely to have used alcohol and/or drugs during sex in the previous six months.

In the multivariate analysis, older participants were more likely to be HIV seropositive than participants under 30 years of age (OR = 3.12; 95% CI = 1.54, 6.33). African-American participants, although there were very few (only 18) in the sample, were nearly four times more likely to be HIV seropositive while controlling for the other demographic variables (OR = 3.79; 95% CI = 1.19, 12.05). Education was found to have a negative association with being HIV seropositive; the more education a person reported, the lower their likelihood of being HIV seropositive (OR = .88; 95% CI = .79, .97). Those who reported exchange sex were twice as likely to be HIV seropositive, but this association was not statistically significant (OR = 1.72; 95% CI = .76, 3.90). (See Table 5.)

The second model incorporated whether someone used alcohol and/or drugs during sex. Those who used alcohol and/or drugs during sex were three times more likely to be HIV seropositive. Demographic factors such as age, over 30 years, African-American race, low income, and low education were also found to be associated with being HIV seropositive. Experience with exchange sex was not found to be associated with being HIV seropositive; however, substance use during sex was strongly associated with HIV seropositivity.

TABLE 4. Regression analyses of risk behaviors by exchange sex, controlling for Latina identity and education.

MULTIPLE LINEAR REGRESSION	Latina		Education		Exchanged Sex		P-Value (F-Test)
	b	Stand Error	b	Stand Error	b	Stand Error	
Number of main partners	-.29+	.16	-.01	.02	.34	.15	2.06
Number of casual partners	2.37	3.32	-.10	.49	7.31*	3.32	2.65*
LOGISTIC REGRESSION	Odds ratio	95% Confidence interval	Odds ratio	95% Confidence interval	Odds ratio	95% Confidence interval	P-value (Chi Sq)
Had sex while high on alcohol or drug	2.71***	1.47-4.99	.94	.85-1.03	3.51***	1.94-6.33	53.42***
Receptive anal w/main partner intercourse	8.76*	1.44-53.33	1.09	.86-1.40	1.37	.32-5.91	8.58*
Receptive anal w/casual partner intercourse	2.08	.71-6.14	1.07	.91-1.25	3.22*	1.17-8.83	9.74*
Unprotected anal receptive sex w/main partner[a]	1.36	.54-3.48	1.00	.87-1.14	.60	.25-1.40	1.51
Unprotected anal receptive sex w/casual partner[a]	.54	.17-1.70	1.12	.93-1.35	.46	.16-1.35	10.10*

[a] Among only those having had anal receptive intercourse, reported intercourse with a condom never or almost never in previous six months.
+ = $p < .1$, * = $p < .05$, *** = $p < .001$

TABLE 5. Logistic regression analysis of HIV seroprevalence by sociodemographic characteristics.

Characteristic	Model 1			Model 2		
	Odds ratio	95% Confidence intervals	P-value	Odds ratio	95% Confidence intervals	P-value
Age Group (30 years or older vs 18-29 years)	3.12	1.54-6.33	<.01	2.71	1.32-5.60	<.01
Female (self-identification vs all others)	.80	.40-1.65	NS	.70	.34-1.45	NS
Race/Ethnicity						
African-American (vs all, controlling for Latinas)	3.79	1.19-12.05	<.05	4.51	1.38-14.76	<.01
Latina vs others	1.50	.59-3.79	NS	1.24	.47-3.23	NS
Country of Birth (US vs others)	.89	.34-2.36	NS	1.11	.40-3.03	NS
Education (used continuously)	.88	.79-.97	<.01	.88	.80-.98	<.05
Annual income (used continuously)	.83	.63-1.10	NS	.80	.60-1.07	NS
No sex in the previous six months (vs reported having sex in the previous six months)	.75	.21-2.63	NS	1.23	.32-4.78	NS
Exchange sex in the previous six months	1.72	.76-3.90	NS	1.46	.64-3.34	NS
Used drugs or alcohol during sex				2.68	1.15-6.28	<.05
Chi Square	31.84		<.0002	37.38		<.0001
−2 Log L	256.93			256.93		

DISCUSSION

This study found many differences between transgendered women who exchanged sex and those who did not. Transgendered women who exchanged sex were more likely to be under thirty years of age, identify as female (especially as a heterosexual female), be Latina (and to have lived in the United States for less than 10 years), and to have less than a high school education. Those who exchanged sex were also less likely to have health insurance or a source of health care. Those who exchanged sex were more likely to have used a condom during receptive and insertive anal intercourse with main and casual sexual partners; however, their greatest HIV risk was unsafe needle use and substance use (especially during sex). Use of alcohol and/or drugs was found to be the greatest behavioral predictor of HIV infection, as was being African-American and having a low socioeconomic status. Exchange sex was not directly associated with HIV infection but it was likely that it was associated with the other factors that related to HIV seroprevalance.

Transgendered women often experience socioeconomic disadvantage, including low income, high unemployment, lower levels of education, and unstable housing (Nemoto et al., 1999), which are likely to contribute to their decision to engage in exchange sex. Additionally, transgendered women experience significant social marginalization (Namaste, 2000; Weinberg, Shaver & Williams, 1999). This is particularly true for newly emigrated Latina transgendered women who may not be acculturated enough to enter many low-level jobs and, at the same time, their transgendered status may limit their employment with many "under-the-table" jobs, thus leaving exchange sex their only viable alternative for income and support (Reback & Lombardi, 2001). Younger transgendered women, particularly those with lower educational attainment, may also have difficulty obtaining legal employment and, similarly, find exchange sex their only option. Furthermore, transitioning from one gender to another at a younger age may result in losing familial support or leaving school (either to support oneself and/or due to harassment experienced in a school setting) and thereby limiting economic opportunities.

Consistent with a previous study (Reback & Lombardi, 2001), the transgendered women in this study who exchanged sex were more likely to report having sex while high on alcohol and/or drugs compared to the transgendered women who did not exchange sex. Additionally, the findings demonstrated that engaging in sex while high was independently associated with increased likelihood of HIV infection. These findings suggest that, as with other populations (Reback, Larkins & Shoptaw, 2004), alcohol and/or drug use may contribute to high-risk sexual practices in transgendered women. Therefore, as with other populations, HIV prevention programs targeting transgendered women should include substance abuse screening protocols as well as linkages to drug treatment services when indicated (Metzger, Navaline & Woody, 1998; Reback, Simon, Bemis & Gatson, 2001).

The participants who exchanged sex were more likely to identify as heterosexual females, while those who did not exchange sex were more likely to identify as transgender and also as heterosexual. This incongruity between their sexual identity, gender identity, and biological sex could explain why they were more likely to use alcohol and/or drugs during sex, as substance use could function as a mechanism to help cope with this disjunction. It is likely that transgendered women want to follow traditional, heterosexual female sexual scripts and thus have their gender and sexual identities reified within their sexual relationships. As such, sex could be a stress provoking activity that is managed through substance use. Similarly, sexually active participants in this study reported a lower likelihood of condom use during receptive anal intercourse with main partners and, again, this finding may be based on their desire to enact sexual scripts coded as traditional, heterosexual female. Finally, sexual activities for these participants may be one of the few ways they can express their gender identity (woman) and sexual identity (heterosexual) and have these identities validated by their male sexual partners (Kammerer, Mason, Connors & Durkee, 2001). Focus groups conducted by the San Francisco Department of Public Health (1997) found that transgendered women reported that the attention they received from male clients was affirming to their gender identity. Health care professionals should address stigma, discrimination and abuse against transgendered women within their practice. Even the most culturally appropriate HIV prevention messages are limited if social barriers against legal employment are so great that transgendered women view exchange sex as one of their few options for employment, or as a means to have both their gender and sexual identities validated by others.

Transgendered women are in need of greater attention in terms of both new research as well as tailored prevention, education, treatment, and support services. These services should address the complex psychological and social factors that may contribute to important risk behaviors by providing educational, occupational, and economic opportunities, as well as linkages to substance abuse treatment services. Most importantly there is the need to understand and support both the gender and sexual identities of these women. Many studies have conceptualized transgendered women as a subset of the "men who have sex with men (MSM)" category. In doing so, these studies, and the interventions and materials that are generated from these studies, are more likely to alienate than educate transgendered women. Gender and sexual identities are often collapsed, even by health care professionals. This is evidenced when transgender, which is a gender identity, is categorized with lesbian, gay and bisexual, which are sexual identities, to create the category of "lesbian, gay, bisexual and transgender" or "LGBT." Most of the transgendered women in this study identified their gender as "female or woman" (56%) and their sexuality as heterosexual (77%). It is important that gender and sexuality are understood as two separate domains when providing HIV prevention messages to transgendered women.

One limitation of this study is its cross-sectional design; these findings are associative and cannot of themselves denote risk. As noted previously, because the findings are based on a convenience sample that included few African-American participants, any conclusions based on race/ethnicity should be interpreted with caution (Simon, Reback & Bemis, 2000). Other limitations include the possibility that, given the sensitivity of many of the questions in the survey, some respondents may have underreported certain risk behaviors. Furthermore, this study interviewed transgendered women that were contacted in a street outreach setting. Thus, transgendered women who only exchange sex in a commercial venue, in their homes or through ads may not have been captured. Further research is needed on different subgroups of transgendered women who exchange sex, specifically those who work in various sex venues. While these findings may not be completely generalizable to other transgendered populations–particularly those that are more affluent or well assimilated–they do provide a profile of those who have had contact with outreach workers and other HIV prevention staff in areas of Los Angeles County where the HIV epidemic has been most severe.

Finally, to determine the true extent of the HIV epidemic in transgendered populations, it is essential to employ gender variables that will capture transgendered individuals while, at the same time, respect their identity. Without these variables, population-based surveys, surveillance databases, as well as other HIV research studies will continue to miss this important risk group.

REFERENCES

Belza, M.J., Llacer A., Mora, R., de la Fuente, L., Castilla, J., Noguer, I., & Canellas, S. (2000). Social characteristics and risk behaviors for HIV in a group of transvestites and male transsexuals engaging in street prostitution (abstract). *Gac Sanit, 14*, 330-337.

Bockting, W.O., Robinson, B.E., & Rosser, B.R.S. (1998). Transgender HIV prevention: a qualitative needs assessment. *AIDS Care, 10*, 505-526.

Bockting, W.O., Rosser, B.R.S., & Scheltema, K. (1999). Transgender HIV prevention: implementation and evaluation of a workshop. *Health Education Research, 14*, 177-183.

Boehmer, U. (2002). Twenty years of public health research: inclusion of lesbian, gay, and transgender populations. *American Journal of Public Health, 92*, 1125-1130.

Boles J. & Elifson, K.W. (1994). The social organization of transvestite prostitution and AIDS. *Social Science Medicine, 39*, 85-93.

Clements-Nolle, K., Marx, R., Guzman, R., & Katz, M. (2001). HIV prevalence, risk behaviors, health care use, and mental health status of transgender persons: implications for public health intervention. *American Journal of Public Health, 91*, 915-921.

Croker, C. (2003). Los Angeles County Department of Health Services, unpublished manuscript and personal communication. December 2003.

Elifson, K.W., Boles, J., Posey, E., Sweat, M., Darrow, W., & Elsea, W. (1993). Male transvestite prostitutes and HIV risk. *American Journal of Public Health, 83*, 260-262.

Gras, M.J., van der Helm, T., Schenk, R., van Doornum, G.J., Coutinho, R.A., & van den Hoek, J.A. (1997). HIV infection and risk behaviour among prostitutes in the Amsterdam streetwalkers' district: indications of raised prevalence of HIV among transvestites (abstract). *Ned Tijdschr Geneesd 141*, 1238-1241.

Harcourt, C., van Beek, I., Heslop, J., McMahon, M., & Donovan, B. (2001). The health and welfare needs of female and transgender street sex workers in new South Wales. *Australian/New Zealand Journal of Public Health, 25*, 84-89.

Inciardi, J.A. & Surratt, H.L. (1997). Male transvestite sex workers and HIV in Rio de Janeiro, Brazil. *Journal of Drug Issues, 27*, 135-146.

Kammerer, N., Mason, T., Connors, M., & Durkee, R. (2001). Transgenders, HIV/AIDS, and substance abuse: from risk group to group prevention. In: *Transgender and HIV: Risks, Prevention, and Care*, 13-38. Walter Bockting & Shelia Kirk, eds. Haworth Press: New York.

Kellogg, T., Clements-Nolle, K., Dilley, J., Katz, M., & McFarland, W. (2001). Incidence of human immunodeficiency virus among male-to-female transgendered persons in San Francisco. *Journal of Acquired Immune Deficiency Syndrome, 28*, 380-384.

Kenagy, G.P. (2002). HIV among transgendered people. *AIDS Care, 14*, 127-134.

Lombardi, E.L., Wilchins, R.A., Priesing, D., & Malouf, D. (2001). Gender violence: transgender experience with violence and discrimination. *Journal of Homosexuality, 42*, 89-101.

Metzger, D.S., Navaline, H. & Woody, G.E. (1998). Drug abuse treatment as AIDS prevention. *Public Health Report, 113*, 97-106.

Modan, B., Goldschmidt, R., Rubinstein, E., Vonsover, A., Zinn, M., Golan, R., Chetrit, A., & Gottlieb-Stematzky, T. (1992). Prevalence of HIV antibodies in transsexual and female prostitutes. *American Journal of Public Health, 82*, 590-592.

Namaste, V.K. (2000). *Invisible lives: the erasure of transsexual and transgendered people*. Chicago: University of Chicago Press.

Nemoto, T., Luke, D., Mamo, L., Ching, A., & Patria, J. (1999). HIV risk behaviours among male-to-female transgenders in comparison with homosexual or bisexual males and heterosexual females. *AIDS Care, 11*, 297-312.

Reback, C.J., Larkins, S., & Shoptaw, S. (2004). Changes in the meaning of sexual risk behaviors among gay and bisexual male methamphetamine abusers before and after drug treatment. *AIDS & Behavior, 8*, 87-98.

Reback, C.J. & Lombardi, E.L. (2001). HIV risk behaviors of male-to-female transgenders in a community-based harm reduction program. In W. Bockting & S. Kirk (Eds). *Transgender and HIV: Risks, Prevention, and Care* (pp. 59-68). New York: The Haworth Press.

Reback, C.J. & Simon, P.A. (2004). The Los Angeles Transgender Health Study: creating a research and community collaboration. In B.P. Bowser, S.I. Miraz, C.J. Reback, & G.F. Lemp (Eds). *Preventing AIDS: Community-Science Collaborations* (pp. 115-131). New York: The Haworth Press.

Reback, C.J., Simon, P.A., Bemis, C.C., & Gatson B. (2001). *The Los Angeles Transgender Health Study: Community Report.* (Report funded by the Universitywide AIDS Research Program.) Los Angeles: Author.

San Francisco Department of Public Health, AIDS Office. (1997). *HIV Prevention And Health Service Needs Of The Transgender Community In San Francisco: Results From Eleven Focus Groups.* San Francisco: San Francisco Department of Public Health, AIDS Office.

Simon, P.A., Reback, C.J., & Bemis, C.C. (2000). HIV prevalence and incidence among male-to-female transsexuals receiving HIV prevention services in Los Angeles County. *AIDS, 14*, 2953-2955.

Spizzichino, L., Zaccarelli, M., Rezza, G., Ippolito, G., Antinori, A., & Gattari, P. (2001). HIV infection among foreign transsexual sex workers in Rome. *Sexually Transmitted Diseases, 28*, 405-411.

Stephens, T., Cozza, S., & Braithwaite, R. (1999). Transsexual orientation in HIV risk behaviours in an adult male prison. *International Journal of STD & AIDS, 10*, 28-31.

Sykes, D.L. (1999). Transgendered people: an "invisible" population. *California HIV/AIDS Update, 12*, 80-85.

Verster, A., Davoli, M., Camposeragna, A., Valeri, C., & Perucci, C.A. (2001). Prevalence of HIV infection and risk behaviour among street prostitutes in Rome, 1997-1998. AIDS Care, 13, 367-372.

Weinberg, M.S., Shaver, F.M., & Williams, C.J. (1999). Gendered sex work in the San Francisco tenderloin. *Archives of Sexual Behavior, 28*, 503-521.

The Connections of Mental Health Problems, Violent Life Experiences, and the Social Milieu of the "Stroll" with the HIV Risk Behaviors of Female Street Sex Workers

Hilary L. Surratt, PhD
Steven P. Kurtz, PhD
Jason C. Weaver, BA
James A. Inciardi, PhD

SUMMARY. This paper examines the connections of mental health, victimization, and sexual risk behaviors among a sample of 278 street-based female sex workers in Miami. Using targeted sampling strategies, drug-using sex workers were recruited into an HIV prevention research program. Data were collected by trained interviewers, and focused on drug use and sexual risk for HIV, childhood abuse, recent victimization, and mental health. More than half of the participants reported histories of

---

Hilary L. Surratt, Steven P. Kurtz, Jason C. Weaver, and James A. Inciardi are all affiliated with the University of Delaware, Center for Drug & Alcohol Studies.

Address correspondence to: Hilary L. Surratt, PhD, 2100 Ponce de Leon Boulevard, Suite 1180, Coral Gables, FL 33134 (E-mail: hsurratt@udel.edu).

This research was supported by HHS Grant #R01-DA13131 from the National Institute on Drug Abuse.

[Haworth co-indexing entry note]: "The Connections of Mental Health Problems, Violent Life Experiences, and the Social Milieu of the 'Stroll' with the HIV Risk Behaviors of Female Street Sex Workers." Surratt, Hilary L. et al. Co-published simultaneously in *Journal of Psychology & Human Sexuality* (The Haworth Press, Inc.) Vol. 17, No. 1/2, 2005, pp. 23-44; and: *Contemporary Research on Sex Work* (ed: Jeffrey T. Parsons) The Haworth Press, Inc., 2005, pp. 23-44. Single or multiple copies of this article are available for a fee from The Haworth Document Delivery Service [1-800-HAWORTH, 9:00 a.m. - 5:00 p.m. (EST). E-mail address: docdelivery@haworthpress.com].

physical (51.1%) or sexual (53.1%) abuse as children, 37.4% were classified with moderate or severe anxiety symptoms, and 52.9% had symptoms of moderate or severe depression. Logistic regression analyses demonstrated significant associations between mental health issues and engagement in recent unprotected vaginal and oral sex. The program development and policy implications of these findings are discussed. *[Article copies available for a fee from The Haworth Document Delivery Service: 1-800-HAWORTH. E-mail address: <docdelivery@haworthpress.com> Website: <http://www.HaworthPress.com>* © *2005 by The Haworth Press, Inc. All rights reserved.]*

KEYWORDS. HIV, sex work, drug abuse, violence, depression

Existing research on female sex workers has demonstrated clear and consistent associations between the sale of sex for money or drugs and an increased risk for HIV and other sexually transmitted infections (STIs) (Cohen & Alexander, 1995; El-Bassel et al., 2001; Paone et al., 1999; Weiner, 1996). However, it is important to emphasize that the ecology of risk tends to vary from one style of sex work to another, and in contrast to popular thinking, female sex workers are an extremely heterogeneous population. They are situated in a myriad of social and environmental contexts, where risk and vulnerability can differ considerably.

Past and current studies suggest that there are many different types of female sex workers, including "call girls" and escorts working in the upper echelons of the sex industry, "in-house" sex workers working in parlors or brothels, "street-walkers" who sell sex for money through sidewalk solicitations, part-timers who supplement their incomes with sex-for-pay, and drug-involved street-based sex workers, the majority of whom shift between sex-for-money and sex-for-drug exchanges as circumstances require (Estébanez et al., 1993; Exner, 1977; Inciardi, 1995; Jones et al., 1998). Although most in this latter group express a preference for commercial solicitation along local "strolls" (i.e., locations where sex workers openly walk the streets soliciting customers), many typically resort to sex-for-drugs exchanges when they have an immediate need for drugs, when money is scarce, and when paying "dates" (customers) are few in number (Inciardi et al., 1993; Inciardi & Surratt, 2001).

Perhaps more important than the particulars of the sexual transaction is a focus on the social location and the related vulnerability of the sex worker herself. Inherent to street sex work is a level of power and control situated far below that of "in-house" or "call girl" type workers. Street-based women typically occupy the "bottom rungs" of the sex-for-pay hierarchy. Concomitant with this position, they are exposed to elevated levels of violence, including rape and assault (Coston & Ross, 1998; El-Bassel et al., 1997; Farley et al., 1998; Kurtz et al., 2004; Surratt et al., 2004; Wenzel, Leake, & Gelberg, 2001), and because of their visibility on the street, the potential for arrest is high (El-Bassel et al., 2001; Jones et al., 1998; McClanahan et al., 1999). Moreover, many are heavy users of cocaine, crack, heroin, and other drugs (Kilbourne et al., 2002; Young, Boyd, & Hubbell, 2000), placing them at high risk for loss of social services and support structures, including family connections and stable housing (Spittal et al., 2003; Valera, Sawyer, & Shiraldi, 2001; Weiner, 1996). Not surprisingly, it is street sex workers who are particularly vulnerable to HIV and other STI exposure (Pyett & Warr, 1997).

With this unstable and often chaotic social milieu as a backdrop, researchers have observed impaired mental health functioning among women enmeshed in street sex exchanges. In contrast to brothel-based sex workers, among whom measures of mental health tend to approximate those of the general population (Chudakov, Ilan, & Belmaker, 2002; Romans et al., 2001), street-based sex workers are more likely to exhibit psychological distress, including symptoms of psychosis and depression (Alegria et al., 1994; El-Bassel et al., 1997; El-Bassel et al., 2001). In a study of Puerto Rican sex workers, for example, Alegria and colleagues (1994) found that 70% of their respondents manifested high levels of depressive symptoms, with rates of depression two times higher than those in a cohort of non-sex working Puerto Rican women. In addition, adolescent female sex workers have demonstrated higher levels of depression, anxiety, alienation, and a less favorable self-concept when compared to samples of non-sex trading delinquents and general population cohorts (Gibson-Ainyette et al., 1988).

It has been suggested, furthermore, that the relationship between sex exchange and psychological distress may be related to increased victimization, including childhood physical and sexual abuse, and adult violence, all of which are frequently reported among female sex workers (El-Bassel et al., 2001; Silbert & Pines, 1983; Surratt et al., 2004; Valera, Sawyer, & Schiraldi, 2001). Early abuse has been independently associated with an increased likelihood of adult drug use, psychological distress, victimization, sexual risk behaviors and involvement in the criminal justice system among non-sex workers (Goodman

& Fallot, 1998; Johnsen & Harlow, 1996; Morrill et al., 2001; Widom & Ames, 1994; Wilsnack et al., 1997; Young, Boyd, & Hubbell, 2000). In addition, elevated rates of adult victimization and psychological distress have been reported among homeless women, female drug abusers, and female sex workers (Farley & Barkan, 1998; Hutton et al., 2001; Reif, Wechsberg, & Dennis, 2001), and these may mediate women's engagement in sexual risk behaviors as fear of partner violence may reduce some women's willingness to challenge, refuse, or negotiate the terms of sexual encounters (Amaro, 1995; Frieze & McHugh, 1992; Heise, 1993).

Going further, studies of drug-using women have repeatedly demonstrated connections between mental health measures, including anxiety, depression and personality disorders, and elevated levels of HIV risk behaviors (Cohen, 1999; Compton et al., 1995; Wechsberg et al., 2003), yet only a few studies have examined these relationships specifically among female sex workers. One longitudinal study of adolescents found not only that depressive symptoms were associated with engagement in sex work, but that an increase in mental health symptoms for depression and suicidality was related to later injection drug use and risky sexual activity (Stiffman et al., 1992). Similarly, studies of adult and adolescent Puerto Rican sex workers found that individuals with high levels of depressive symptoms more often reported inconsistent condom use with their sexual partners (Alegria et al., 1994; Burgos et al., 1999).

Among street sex workers who are drug-involved, risky sexual behaviors increase. In addition to sexual contact with multiple partners, condom use among crack using sex workers tends to be low and inconsistent with both oral and vaginal sex, with both paid and private partners (Jones et al., 1998; Pyett & Warr, 1997; Rhodes & Donoghoe, 1994; Weiner, 1996).

In spite of the physical and psychological vulnerability resulting from street-based violence and unstable living conditions, studies which describe the associations between mental health functioning and engagement in sexual risk behaviors among chronic drug-using sex workers are noticeably absent.

Within this context, this study examined the prevalence of specific mental health problems among a cohort of drug-involved, street-based female sex workers in Miami, Florida, by collecting standardized measures of current symptom level information on depression, anxiety, and traumatic stress among this understudied population, and investigated the associations between mental health status and sexual risk taking behaviors among women located in an environment of scarce material resources, homelessness, and violent victimization. In this regard, this analysis was undertaken to explore the following questions: (1) What is the extent of childhood abuse, adult victimization and symptomatology for depression, anxiety and traumatic stress in a sample of street-based, drug-involved female sex workers?; and (2) Within this sample, is there an association between current mental health symptoms, violent victimization in childhood and adulthood, and engagement in sexual risk behaviors for HIV and other sexually transmitted infections, and if so, what is the nature of this association?

METHODS

Participants and Procedures

The data for this study were drawn from a larger, ongoing intervention trial designed to test the relative effectiveness of two alternative HIV and hepatitis prevention protocols–the National Institute on Drug Abuse (NIDA) "Standard Intervention" (designed for a myriad of drug-using populations) and a new Sex Worker-Focused Intervention (developed specifically to reduce the risky drug use and sexual behaviors of street-based female sex workers). The Standard Intervention, developed by NIDA researchers and grantees (Wechsberg et al., 1997), includes individual pretest counseling covering such topics as HIV disease, transmission routes, risky drug-using behaviors, unsafe sexual practices, rehearsal of condom use, disinfection of injection equipment, and rehearsal of needle/syringe cleaning. The Sex Worker-Focused Intervention is unique in that it was developed by the authors of this paper with input from active sex workers. In addition to the topics covered in the NIDA Standard Intervention, it addresses issues of special relevance to the target population, including the violent encounters and the barriers to safe sex experienced by street sex workers (Surratt et al. 2004).

Eligible participants were defined as women ages 18 to 49 who have: (a) traded sex for money or drugs at least 3 times in the past 30 days; and, (b) used heroin and/or cocaine 3 or more times a week in the past 30 days. Although it has been argued in the literature that "sex work" and "sex exchange" are behaviorally different phenomena (Cohen & Alexander, 1995), prior research in Miami combined with information from key informants suggest that these distinctions are less clear in the neighborhoods and "strolls" where study participants are recruited. Nearly all of the drug-involved street-based sex workers in Miami engage in sex-for-money and sex-for-drug exchanges as opportunities arise.

Participants in the study were located for recruitment through traditional targeted sampling strategies (Watters & Biernacki, 1989), which are especially useful for studying hard-to-reach populations. As opposed to "snowball sampling" which begins with one or more initial contacts or starting points and expands through a chain referral process (Inciardi, 1986; Waldorf, 1973), targeted sampling is a more purposeful, systematic method by which specified populations within geographical districts are identified, and detailed plans are designed to recruit adequate numbers of cases within each of the target areas. Similar strategies have been used successfully in recent years in studies of injection and other out-of-treatment drug users (Coyle et al., 1991; Carlson et al., 1994; Braunstein, 1993).

A unique aspect of the project's sampling plan is the use of active sex workers as client recruiters. The effectiveness of indigenous client recruiters in drug abuse and HIV prevention research has been well documented (Inciardi, Surratt, & McCoy, 1997; Latkin, 1998; Levy & Fox, 1998; Wiebel, 1990, 1993). Because active sex workers do the recruiting of study participants, and because of their membership in the target population, they know of many locations on and off the primary strolls where potential participants can be found. In addition, sex worker recruiters are more likely to have familiarity with drug user networks, drug "copping areas" and markets; they typically approach potential clients with culturally appropriate language, dress, and methods; and their "insider status" helps to build the trust and confidence necessary for successful outreach and recruitment.

Client recruiters made contact with potential participants in various street locations to explain the nature and procedures of the study. For those interested in participation, recruiters conducted pre-screening interviews to determine eligibility. Those meeting project eligibility requirements were scheduled for appointments at the project intervention center, where they were re-screened by project staff members. After eligibility was confirmed, informed consent was obtained and urine testing was conducted for cocaine and opiates. The interview process took approximately ninety minutes to complete. Interviews were conducted in Spanish by bilingual field staff for the few participants who were not fluent in English. All study procedures were reviewed and approved by the University of Delaware's Institutional Review Board.

Study recruitment began in March 2001, and through late 2003, more than 600 eligible clients had been recruited, enrolled, and interviewed.

Supplementary support was awarded by the funding agency in mid-2002 to conduct mental health assessments and to provide case management services and referrals for women enrolled in the larger study. As such, mental health data are available on 278 street-based sex workers, who are the focus of this analysis.

Measures

Interviews were conducted using a standardized data collection instrument based primarily on the NIDA Risk Behavior Assessment (Dowling-Guyer et al., 1994; Needle et al., 1995; Weatherby et al., 1994) and the Georgia State University Prostitution Inventory (Elifson, 1990). This instrument captures demographic information, health status, and treatment history, as well as lifetime and 30 day measures of drug use frequency and sexual risk behaviors. The following key measures of mental health and trauma were also utilized:

Childhood Trauma Questionnaire (short form) (Bernstein et al., 1994). The CTQ-SF assesses the prevalence and extent of childhood physical, sexual and emotional abuse, as well physical and emotional neglect. The CTQ-SF is a 28-item instrument that uses a 5-item Likert scale ranging from 1 (Never True) to 5 (Very Often True), thereby capturing severity data on abuse and neglect history unavailable with categorical measures. Summary subscale scores range from 5 to 25 and are classified as none, minimal, moderate or severe according to criteria set by the authors of the scale. Severe sexual and physical abuse classifications required scores of 13 or higher, while severe emotional abuse required a score of at least 16. Only abuse subscales are reported in this paper. The alpha reliability coefficients for this sample were as follows: 0.87 (emotional abuse), 0.89 (physical abuse), and 0.96 (sexual abuse).

Beck Depression Inventory-II (Beck, Steer, & Brown, 1996) contains 21 items to assess the presence and severity of symptoms of depression over the preceding two week period, and is consistent with DSM-IV criteria. A four-point rating on 19 of the items and a seven-point rating on two items are summed to yield a single score classified as minimal (0-13), mild (14-19), moderate (20-28), or severe (29-63). In this sample, the alpha reliability coefficient for the depression scale was 0.92.

Beck Anxiety Inventory (Beck & Steer, 1993) contains 21 items to assess the presence and severity of symptoms of anxiety over the preceding one week period, including subjective, somatic and panic-related symptoms. A four-point rating on each of the 21 items is summed to yield a single score classified as minimal (0-7), mild (8-15), moderate (16-25), or severe (26-63). In this sample, the alpha reliability coefficient for the anxiety scale was 0.92.

Traumatic Stress Index (Dennis, 2003). Based on the Civilian Mississippi PTSD scale (Kulka et al., 1991), this scale consists of 12 yes/no items assessing the presence of symptoms of stress disorders related to past trauma over a 3 month period, but does not distinguish PTSD, Acute Stress Disorder or other stress disorders. The summary score yeilds a classification of none (0), low (1-4) or acute (5-12). The alpha reliability coefficient for the traumatic stress scale in this sample was 0.86.

Data Analysis

Descriptive statistics were compiled on demographic characteristics, drug use, experiences of childhood and adult victimization, symptoms of depression, anxiety and traumatic stress, as well as sexual risk behaviors of the participants. Bivariate logistic regression analyses were then conducted to examine the relationship between sexual risk behaviors for HIV, specifically unprotected vaginal and oral contact, and each of the following possible independent predictors: age, race/ethnicity, current homelessness, current alcohol use, current marijuana use, current cocaine use, current crack use, current heroin use, number of lifetime sexual partners, number of sexual partners in the past thirty days, history of sexually transmitted infections, victimization by customers or "dates" in the past month and past year, victimization by any perpetrator in past three months, history of childhood physical, emotional and sexual abuse, and symptoms of depression, anxiety and traumatic stress. Significant factors in the bivariate analyses were subsequently entered into a multivariate stepwise logistic regression model to examine their combined prediction of engagement in unprotected vaginal sex, while a separate model examined engagement in unprotected oral sex. Victimization by customers or "dates" in the past month and past year, victimization by any perpetrator in past three months, history of childhood physical, emotional and sexual abuse, and symptoms of depression, anxiety and traumatic stress were included as explanatory variables in order to investigate the effects of victimization and psychological functioning on sexual risk taking behaviors. All analyses were conducted using the Statistical Package for the Social Sciences (SPSS) v.11.5.1 for Windows.

RESULTS

The participants ranged from 18 to 49 years of age, with a mean of 35.2 years (Table 1). In terms of race/ethnicity, the majority (70.9%) were African-American. The living situation of the sex workers was typically unstable, with 38.5% reporting that they considered themselves to be homeless. While the remainder were sheltered, they were often precariously housed in nightly hotels, temporary public shelters, rooming houses, or the homes of acquaintances. Only 24% reported having their own stable living space. More than half of the sample (54.0%) failed to complete their high school education, and very few had legal employment (6.8%). The majority had incomes of less than $1,000 per month, primarily from sex work, but also from other illegal

TABLE 1. Demographic Characteristics of 278 Female Sex Workers in Miami, Florida

Age	
18-24	14.4%
25-34	28.0%
35-39	24.1%
40+	33.5%
Mean	35.2
Race/Ethnicity	
African-American	70.9%
White-Anglo	12.6%
Latina	14.4%
Other	2.2%
Education	
Less than High School	54.0%
High School	28.0%
More than High School	18.0%
Monthly Income	
Less than $500	18.0%
$500-999	34.2%
$1,000-1,999	24.5%
$2,000+	23.3%
Currently Homeless	38.5%

activities, spouse or family members, and welfare or public assistance programs.

As illustrated in Table 2, the drug use and sex work histories of the participants were substantial. The participants were typically poly-drug users, and reports of past month activity indicated that alcohol and crack-cocaine were the substances most widely used (79.4% and 68.0%, respectively). A history of drug injection was reported by 19.8% of the women.

The sex work careers of the participants spanned an average of 13.4 years, with a mean of over 1,400 lifetime sexual partners. Current (past month) sex work activities most often included vaginal and oral sexual contacts, with a mean of 18.2 sexual partners. Of significance was the finding that 18.7% of the participants tested positive for HIV, 47.5% tested positive for hepatitis B, and 18.7% tested positive for hepatitis C (data not shown).

TABLE 2. Drug Use and Sex Work Histories Among 278 Female Street Sex Workers in Miami, Florida

Percent Currently Using	
Alcohol	79.4%
Marijuana	65.2%
Crack-cocaine	68.0%
Cocaine	49.3%
Heroin	18.4%
Mean Years of Sex Work	13.4
Mean Number of Sex Partners	
Lifetime	1,470.8
Mean Number of Sex Partners	
Past 30 Days	18.2
% Reporting Past Month[1]	
Unprotected Vaginal Sex	57.1%
Unprotected Oral Sex	65.7%

[1] n = 273, participating in past month vaginal sex;
n = 216, participating in past month oral sex.

Drug involvement and street-based sex work tended to expose women to violent episodes in their daily lives, often deepening and extending patterns of victimization from childhood. Interesting in this regard were the historical self-reports of trauma experienced by the participants as children. As indicated in Table 3, the prevalence of childhood abuse in this sample was extremely elevated. Similarly, 36.0% of the women reported some violent encounter while engaging in sex work in the past year, most frequently being "ripped off" (being forced to give up money that was paid for sex), beaten, threatened, or raped by a customer or date. When individuals other than "dates" were

TABLE 3. Victimization and Mental Health Among 278 Female Street Sex Workers in Miami, Florida

Childhood Victimization	
Emotional Abuse	64.7%
Physical Abuse	51.1%
Sexual Abuse	53.1%
% Any Violent Encounter	
In Past 3 Months	71.2%
% Violent "Date" Encounter	
In Past Month	16.9%
In Past Year	36.0%
% Depression Symptoms	
Minimal/Mild	47.1%
Moderate/Severe	52.9%
% Anxiety Symptoms	
Minimal/Mild	62.6%
Moderate/Severe	37.4%
% Traumatic Stress Symptoms	
None	7.2%
Low	23.6%
Acute	69.2%

considered as perpetrators of violence, the percentage reporting a violent encounter (physical, sexual or emotional) in the past three months jumped to 71.2%. Typically, these perpetrators were boyfriends, drug dealers, or other street people, but victimization by police officers and relatives was reported as well.

Within the context of these violent life experiences, self-report mental health inventories administered to the participants revealed that significant proportions of the sample were affected by psychological issues, specifically anxiety, depression, and traumatic stress. Over one-third of the women assessed were classified with moderate or severe anxiety symptoms (37.4%), more than one-half had symptoms of moderate or severe depression (52.9%), and 69.2% had symptoms of acute traumatic stress.

As noted earlier in Table 2 above, 57.1% of the participants reported unprotected vaginal sex in the past month. Table 4 presents the results of the bivariate and multivariate logistic regression analyses conducted in order to assess the potential effects of trauma, victimization and mental health issues on this specific sexual risk behavior, along with other possible predictors as well. In the bivariate models, the factors significantly related to engaging in unprotected vaginal sex included homelessness (p = .009), moderate/severe depression (p = .004), moderate/severe anxiety (p = .000), acute traumatic stress (p = .019), severe child sexual abuse (p = .011), and any victimization over the past three months (p = .01). When all of these independent predictors were included in a multivariate model, only homelessness (p = .037) and moderate/severe anxiety (p = .000) remained significant. Accordingly, homeless women were 1.7 times more likely than non-homeless women to engage in unprotected vaginal sex, while women with moderate to severe anxiety were 2.7 times more likely to report vaginal sex without a condom than women classified with minimal or mild anxiety.

Table 5 displays the results of bivariate and multivariate logistic models predicting engagement in unprotected oral sex in the past month. Again, bivariate modeling indicated that moderate/severe depression (p = .026), moderate/severe anxiety (p = .018) and moderate childhood physical abuse (.033) were significant predictors of unprotected oral-genital contact in the past month. The full multivariate model found moderately to severely depressed sex workers more than 2 times as likely to engage in unprotected oral sex compared to their non- or minimally-depressed counterparts, and those with moderate physical abuse histories 4 times more likely to engage in unprotected oral sex than those not experiencing childhood physical abuse.

TABLE 4. Predictors of Unprotected Vaginal Sex in Logistic Regression Models Among 273 Female Sex Workers in Miami, Florida

Bivariate Predictors[1]	Regression Coeff.	Odds Ratio	95% CI	Sign. Level
Homelessness[2]	.681	1.976	(1.19, 3.29)	.009
Moderate/Severe Depression[2]	.709	2.032	(1.25, 3.31)	.004
Moderate/Severe Anxiety[2]	1.054	2.868	(1.69, 4.87)	.000
Childhood Sexual Abuse[2]				
Minimal	.383	1.467	(.442, 4.86)	.531
Moderate	.634	1.886	(.918, 3.87)	.084
Severe	.723	2.060	(1.18, 3.60)	.011
Any Victimization in Past 3 Months[2]	.698	2.009	(1.18, 3.42)	.010
Traumatic Stress[2]				
Low	.494	1.639	(0.58, 4.64)	.353
Acute	1.156	3.176	(1.21, 8.34)	.019
Multivariate Predictors				
Moderate/Severe Anxiety[2]	.963	2.619	(1.53, 4.49)	.000
Homelessness[2]	.558	1.748	(1.03, 2.96)	.037

[1] Non significant predictors included age, race, current alcohol use, current marijuana use, current crack use, current cocaine use, current heroin use, victimization by "dates" in past month, victimization by "dates" in past year, number of lifetime sexual partners, number of current sexual partners, STI history, childhood physical abuse, and childhood emotional abuse.
[2] Reference category is "no."

DISCUSSION

Although many of the current discussions of the public health risks associated with sex work focus on HIV and other sexually transmitted infections (UNAIDS 2004), there is a considerable body of literature documenting significant levels of other public health problems that have been experienced by women in the sex industry, including childhood abuse, adult victimization, and symptomatology for depression, anxiety, and other mental health problems (Baldwin, 1993; Belton,

TABLE 5. Predictors of Unprotected Oral Sex in Logistic Regression Models Among 216 Female Sex Workers in Miami, Florida

Bivariate Predictors[1]	Regression Coeff.	Odds Ratio	95% CI	Sign. Level
Moderate/Severe Depression[2]	.646	1.908	(1.08, 3.37)	.026
Moderate/Severe Anxiety[2]	.728	2.071	(1.13, 3.79)	.018
Childhood Physical Abuse[2]				
Minimal	−.609	.544	(.244, 1.21)	.136
Moderate	1.384	3.990	(1.12, 14.22)	.033
Severe	.085	1.088	(.544, 2.18)	.811
Multivariate Predictors				
Moderate/Severe Depression[2]	.756	2.129	(1.17, 3.89)	.014
Childhood Physical Abuse[2]				
Minimal	−.728	.483	(.212, 1.10)	.083
Moderate	1.406	4.078	(1.13, 14.70)	.032
Severe	−.113	.893	(.434, 1.84)	.758

[1] Non significant predictors included age, race, homelessness, current alcohol use, current marijuana use, current crack use, current cocaine use, current heroin use, victimization by "dates" in past month, victimization by "dates" in past year, any victimization in past 3 months, traumatic stress, number of lifetime sexual partners, number of current sexual partners, STI history, childhood sexual abuse, and childhood emotional abuse.
[2] Reference category is "no."

1992; Farley & Barkan, 1998; Giobbe, 1990; Mahan, 1996). In this study of drug-involved, female sex workers recruited from the streets of Miami, Florida, a clear majority of the participants reported these violent incidents and mental health problems.

Of the 278 sex workers interviewed, 53.1% reported sexual abuse as children. This prevalence is not unlike that found in other research on female drug abusers, who are not necessarily sex workers. For example, in a study of 181 drug using women in San Antonio who completed the

Childhood Trauma Questionnaire, 60% reported sexual abuse and 55% reported physical abuse (Medrano et al., 2003). Similarly, among 60 recovering chemically dependent women living in a residential treatment facility, 43% experienced some kind of unwanted childhood sexual experiences with relatives, 51.6% with persons outside of the family, and overall, 68% had been sexually abused sometime in childhood (Teets, 1995). Slightly lower figures were reported in a study of 1,478 community recruited, drug using female partners of injection drug users in Los Angeles, San Diego, and Boston, in that 39.5% had experienced some sort of sexual abuse in childhood (Freeman, Collier, & Parillo, 2002).

Given the literature supporting the relationships between childhood sexual abuse and later drug use (Brabant, Forsyth, & LeBlanc, 1997; Medrano et al., 1999; Widom, Weiler, & Cottler, 1999), and between childhood sexual abuse and adult careers in sex work (Boyle et al., 1997; Jeffreys, 1997; Maher, 1997), one might expect that the 53.1% prevalence of childhood sexual abuse reported in this study should be even higher, given that the sampled women were both drug users and sex workers. In all likelihood, the prevalence of childhood sexual abuse was underreported by the women studied, for two reasons. First, the research interview occurred during the first contact that participants had with the project staff. As such, the sex workers were in unfamiliar surroundings, and some may have been unwilling to discuss extremely traumatic events from their childhood. Second, and perhaps more notably, informal discussions with project participants found that many were uncertain as to what sexual "abuse" actually was. As young children, some were unaware that sexual contacts without penetration were "sex," and for many others, coercion in the absence of physical force was not necessarily viewed as abuse. This finding has been reported elsewhere in the literature (Farley & Barkan, 1998).

Violent victimization during the course of sex work was commonplace, in that 71.2% of the women in this study had been victimized during the three-month period prior to recruitment into the study. This proportion was considerably higher than that seen in other studies. For example, a study of 113 street based sex workers in New York City found that 32.1% had suffered physical or sexual abuse in the past year (El-Bassel et al., 2001), and a British study of 115 women found that 50% had been victimized by a commercial customer in the prior 6 months (Church et al., 2001). Perhaps most significantly, a recent National Violence Against Women survey sponsored by the National Institute of Justice and the Centers for Disease Control and Prevention placed the percentage of women in the general population experiencing rape or physical assault in the past 12 months at 0.3% and 1.9%, respectively (Tjaden & Thoennes, 1998). In this analysis of drug-involved sex workers, the rates of violence from dates and other perpetrators are many times higher, supporting the contention that female sex workers are enmeshed in a social milieu wherein violence is commonplace and victimization is expected. These data provide a context to understand the elevated rates of acute traumatic stress observed in this sample of drug-involved sex workers.

This study also documented elevated prevalence rates of current depression and anxiety among the sample of street-based female sex workers. These data are supported by similar studies reporting high levels of past year depressive symptoms in 64% to 70% of street sex workers (Alegria et al., 1994; Burgos et al., 1999), and well exceed the rates of current depression in both incarcerated women (10%) and women in the general population (5% to 9%) (Hutton et al., 2001). Moreover, these levels of depressive symptoms are significantly higher than those of other female drug users who are not necessarily sex workers. For example, in a study of 420 African American female, out-of-treatment drug users in St. Louis, only 11% reported depression during the past month (Johnson, Williams, & Cottler, 2002).

The drug-involved sex workers from which the women in this study were sampled represent one of the most highly marginalized populations in the Miami area. All are indigent, and given their drug use, combined with the shifting and precarious nature of their resources, health, safety, and social ties, it is not surprising that many reported being homeless at the time of study recruitment. The finding that homelessness was a significant predictor of recent unprotected vaginal sex is also not unexpected, considering the effects of marginalization and economic deprivation on the women's need to engage in sex work as a survival mechanism (Inciardi, 1995). As such, this analysis has identified key individual and contextual factors that increase street sex workers' vulnerability to sexual risks. However, although 18.7% of the women tested positive for HIV infection, an interesting finding in these data is the lack of an association between mental health symptoms, homelessness, or economic circumstances, and HIV seropositivity. Focus groups and in-depth interviews with many of the sex workers as well as discussions with key informants in the street culture, however, suggested a plausible explanation. It would appear that although only 38.5% reported being homeless at the time of recruitment into the study, cycling in and out of homelessness is a lifestyle pattern experienced by an overwhelming majority of the drug-involved, female sex workers in this sample. As such, sexual risks tended to increase during periods of homelessness, and it is likely that at one point or another, virtually all of the women in the sample were at increased risk for infection. In other words, all of the women, whether homeless or not at the time of their interview, were at comparable risk for HIV over time.

During the course of this study, arrangements were made for participants to receive the results of their mental health assessments, and referrals for services, if necessary, and almost three-fourths (73%) of the women returned for this appointment. Using detailed locator information collected at the first interview, staff were often able to re-contact participants through telephone or mailings for follow-up appointments. When these strategies failed, field staff tracked participants in the streets and other locales they were known to frequent. Although almost one-third required no referral, another 30% either refused the referral or stated that they were already in some form of counseling. Of the 34% who accepted the referral, all but 3 failed to follow through with the referral recommendations. The reasons for this non-compliance were many: services required payment or insurance; the majority of the service providers required that the sex workers produce identification, and most of the women either had none or were unwilling to show it; few of the women had access to the necessary transportation; many were afraid of being labeled as "crazy"; and almost all expressed a dislike for mental health professionals.

Given that this population is in great need of mental health services, these observations suggest a number of program development and policy changes that may assist in effectively reaching female sex workers. First, mental health services need to be integrated into other types of locations where drug-involved sex workers are more likely to visit, such as shelters and substance abuse treatment programs. Second, services need to be sensitive to the barriers faced by this population, such as providing transportation and not requiring identification. Third, and perhaps most importantly, mental health service providers need to create an environment where sex workers and other marginalized populations are treated with respect and are cared for in a non-judgmental manner. From a public health point of view, opportunities for mental health treatment for this population, as well as substance abuse treatment, must be integrated into prevention programs for sex workers in order to effectively decrease risk for HIV and other sexually transmitted infections.

REFERENCES

Alegria, M., Vera, M., Freeman, D. H., Robles, R., Santos, M. C., & Rivera, C. L. (1994). HIV infection, risk behaviors, and depressive symptoms among Puerto Rican sex workers. *American Journal of Public Health, 84*(12), 200-202.

Amaro, H. (1995). Love, sex, and power: Considering women's realities in HIV prevention. *American Psychologist, 50*(6), 437-447.

Baldwin, M. A. (1992). Split at the root: Prostitution and feminist discourses of law reform. *Yale Journal of Law and Feminism, 5,* 47-120.

Beck, A. T., & Steer, R. A. (1993). *Beck anxiety inventory manual.* San Antonio, TX: The Psychological Corporation.

Beck, A. T., Steer, R. A., & Brown, G. K. (1996). *Beck depression inventory manual* (2nd ed.). San Antonio, TX: The Psychological Corporation.

Belton, R. (1992, October 22). *Prostitution as traumatic reenactment.* Los Angeles.

Bernstein, D. P., Fink, L., Handelsman, L., Foote, J., Lovejoy, M., Wenzel, K., Sapareto, E., & Ruggiero, J. (1994). Initial reliability and validity of a new retrospective measure of child abuse and neglect. *American Journal of Psychiatry, 151*(8), 1132-1136.

Bourgois, P. (1995). *In search of respect: Selling crack in el barrio.* New York: Cambridge University Press.

Boyle, F. M., Glennon, S., Najman, J. M., Turrell, G., Western, J. S., & Wood, C. (1997). *The sex industry: A survey of sex workers in Queensland, Australia.* Aldershot, England: Ashgate Publishing Limited.

Brabant, S., Forsyth, C. J., & LeBlanc, J. B. (1997). Childhood sexual trauma and substance misuse: A pilot study. *Substance Use and Misuse, 32*(10), 1417-1431.

Braunstein, M. S. (1993). Sampling a hidden population: Noninstitutionalized drug users. *AIDS Education and Prevention, 5*(2), 131-139.

Burgos, M., Richter, D. L., Reininger, B., Coker, A. L., Saunders, R., Alegria, M., & Vera, M. (1999). Street-based female adolescent Puerto Rican sex workers: Contextual issues and health needs. *Family and Community Health, 22*(2), 59-71.

Carlson, R. G., Wang, J., Siegal, H. A., Falck, R. S., & Guo, J. (1994). An ethnographic approach to targeted sampling: Problems and solutions in AIDS prevention research among injection drug and crack-cocaine users. *Human Organization, 53,* 279-286.

Chitwood, D. D., Rivers, J. E., & Inciardi, J. A. (1996). *The American pipe dream: Crack cocaine and the inner city.* Fort Worth, TX: Harcourt Brace College Publishers.

Chudakov, B., Ilan, K., & Belmaker, R. H. (2002). The motivation and mental health of sex workers. *Journal of Sex & Marital Therapy, 28,* 305-315.

Church, S., Henderson, M., Barnard, M., & Hart, G. (2001). Violence by clients towards female prostitutes in different work settings: Questionnaire survey. *British Medical Journal, 322*(7285), 524-525.

Cohen, E. D. (1999). An exploratory attempt to distinguish subgroups among crack-abusing African-American women. *Journal of Addictive Diseases, 18*(3), 41-54.

Cohen, J. B., & Alexander, P. (1995). Female sex workers: Scapegoats in the AIDS epidemic. In O'Leary A. & Jemmott L. S. (Eds.), *Women at risk, issues in the primary prevention of AIDS* (pp. 195-215). New York: Plenum Press.

Compton, W. B., Cottler, L. B., Shillington, A. M., & Price, R. K. (1995). Is antisocial personality disorder associated with increased HIV risk behaviors in cocaine users? *Drug and Alcohol Dependence, 37*(1), 37-43.

Coston, C. T. M., & Ross, L. E. (1998). Criminal victimization of prostitutes: Empirical support for the lifestyle/exposure model. *Journal of Crime and Justice, 21*(1), 53-70.

Coyle, S. L., Boruch, R. F., & Turner, C. F. (Eds.). (1991). *Evaluating AIDS prevention programs* (expanded ed.). Washington, DC: National Academy Press.

Dowling-Guyer, S., Johnson, M., Fisher, D., Needle, R., Watters, J. et al. (1994). Reliability of drug-users' self-reported HIV risk behavior and validity of self-reported recent drug use. *Assessment, 1*(4), 383-392.

El-Bassel, N., Schilling, R. F., Irwin, K. L., Faruque, S., Gilbert, L., Von Bargen, J., Serrano, Y., & Edlin, B. R. (1997). Sex trading and psychological distress among women recruited from the streets of Harlem. *American Journal of Public Health, 87*(1), 66-70.

El-Bassel, N., Simoni, J. M., Cooper, D. K., Gilbert, L., & Schilling, R. (2001). Sex trading and psychological distress among women on methadone. *Psychology of Addictive Behaviors, 15*(3), 177-184.

Elifson, K. W. (1990). *The Georgia state prostitution inventory.* Atlanta, GA.

Estébanez, P., Fitch, K., & Nájera, R. (1993). HIV and female sex workers. *Bulletin of the World Health Organization, 71*(3/4), 397-412.

Exner, J. E., Wylie, J., Leura, A., & Parrill, T. (1977). Some psychological characteristics of prostitutes. *Journal of Personality Assessment, 41*(5), 474-485.

Farley, M., Baral, I., Kiremire, M., & Sezgin, U. (1998). Prostitution in five countries: Violence and post-traumatic stress disorder. *Feminism & Psychology, 8*(4), 405-426.

Farley, M., & Barkan, H. (1998). Prostitution, violence and posttraumatic stress disorder. *Women & Health, 27*(3), 37-49.

Freeman, R. C., Collier, K., & Parillo, K. M. (2002). Early life sexual abuse as a risk factor for crack cocaine use in a sample of community-recruited women at high risk for illicit drug use. *American Journal of Drug and Alcohol Abuse, 28*(1), 109-132.

Frieze, I. H., & McHugh, M. C. (1992). Power and influence strategies in violent and nonviolent marriages. *Psychology of Women Quarterly, 16*, 449-465.

Gibson-Ainyette, I., Templer, D. I., Brown, R., & Veaco, L. (1988). Adolescent female prostitutes. *Archives of Sexual Behavior, 17*(2), 431-438.

Giobbe, E., Harrigan, M., Ryan, J., & Gamache, D. (1990). *Prostitution: A matter of violence against women: Whisper,* 3060 Bloomington Ave., S., MN 55407.

Goodman, L. A., & Fallot, R. D. (1998). HIV risk-behavior in poor urban women with serious mental disorders: Association with childhood physical and sexual abuse. *American Journal of Orthopsychiatry, 68*(1), 73-83.

Heise, L., & Elias, C. (1995). Transforming AIDS prevention to meet women's needs: A focus on developing countries. *Social Science and Medicine, 40*, 931-943.

Hutton, H. E., Treisman, G. J., Hunt, W. R., Fishman, M., Kendig, N., Swetz, A., & Lyketsos, C. G. (2001). HIV risk behaviors and their relationship to posttraumatic stress disorder among women prisoners. *Psychiatric Services, 52*(4), 508-513.

Inciardi, J. A. (1986). *The war on drugs: Heroin, cocaine, crime, and public policy.* Mountain View, CA: Mayfield Publishing Company.

Inciardi, J. A. (1992). *The war on drugs II: The continuing epic of heroin, cocaine, crack, crime, AIDS, and public policy.* Mountain View, CA: Mayfield Publishing Company.

Inciardi, J. A. (1995). Crack, crack house sex, and HIV risk. *Archives of Sexual Behavior, 24*(3), 249-269.

Inciardi, J. A., Lockwood, D., & Pottieger, A. E. (1993). *Women and crack-cocaine.* New York: Macmillan.

Inciardi, J. A., & Surratt, H. L. (2001). Drug use, street crime and sex-trading among cocaine-dependent women: Implications for public health and criminal justice policy. *Journal of Psychoactive Drugs, 33*(4), 379-389.

Inciardi, J. A., Surratt, H. L., & McCoy, H. V. (1997). Establishing an HIV/AIDS intervention program for street drug users in a developing nation. *Journal of Drug Issues, 27*, 173-193.

Jeffreys, S. (1997). *The idea of prostitution.* North Melbourne, Australia: Spinifex Press Pty Ltd.

Johnsen, L. W., & Harlow, L. L. (1996). Childhood sexual abuse linked with adult substance use, victimization, and AIDS-risk. *AIDS Education and Prevention, 8*(1), 44-57.

Johnson, S. D., Cunningham-Williams, R. M., & Cottler, L. B. (2003). A tripartite of HIV-risk for African American women: The intersection of drug use, violence, and depression. *Drug and Alcohol Dependence, 70*, 169-175.

Jones, D. L., Irwin, K. L., Inciardi, J. A., Bowser, B., Schilling, R., Word, C., Evans, P., Faruque, S., Mccoy, H. V., & Edlin, B. R. (1998). The high-risk sexual practices of crack-smoking sex workers recruited from the streets of three American cities. *Sexually Transmitted Diseases, 25*(4), 187-193.

Kilbourne, A. M., Herndon, B., Anderson, R. M., Wenzel, S. L., & Gelberg, L. (2002). Psychiatric symptoms, health services, and HIV risk factors among homeless women. *Journal of Health Care for the Poor and Underserved, 13*, 49-65.

Kurtz, S. P., Surratt, H. L., Inciardi, J. A., & Kiley, M. C. (2004). Sex work and "date" violence. *Violence Against Women, 10*(4), 357-385.

Latkin, C. A. (1998). Outreach in natural settings: The use of peer leaders for HIV prevention among drug users' networks. *Public Health Reports, 113*(Suppl.1), 151-159.

Levy, J. A., & Fox, S. E. (1998). The outreach-assisted model of partner notification with IDUs. *Public Health Reports, 113*(Suppl.1), 160-169.

Mahan, S. (1996). *Crack cocaine, crime, and women: Legal, social, and treatment issues* (Vol. 4). Thousand Oaks, CA: Sage Publications.

Maher, L. (1997). *Sexed work: Gender, race and resistance in a Brooklyn drug market.* New York: Oxford University Press.

McClanahan, S. F., McClelland, G. M., Abram, K. M., & Teplin, L. A. (1999). Pathways into prostitution among female jail detainees and their implications for mental health services. *Psychiatric Services, 50,* 1606-1613.

Medrano, M. A., Desmond, D. P., Zule, W. A., & Hatch, J. P. (1999). Histories of childhood trauma and the effects of risky HIV behaviors in a sample of women drug users. *American Journal of Drug and Alcohol Abuse, 25*(4), 593-606.

Medrano, M. A., Hatch, J. P., Zule, W. A., & Desmond, D. P. (2003). Childhood trauma and adult prostitution behavior in a multiethnic heterosexual drug-using population. *American Journal of Drug and Alcohol Abuse, 29*(2), 463-487.

Morrill, A. C., Kasten, L., Urato, M., & Larson, M. J. (2001). Abuse, addiction, and depression as pathways to sexual risk in women and men with a history of substance abuse. *Journal of Substance Abuse, 13,* 169-184.

Needle, R., Weatherby, N. L., Brown, B. S., Booth, R., Williams, M. L., Watters, J. K., Andersen, M., Chitwood, D. D., Fisher, D. G., Cesari, H., & Braunstein, M. (1995). Reliability of self reported HIV risk behaviors of drug users. *Psychology of Addictive Behaviors, 9,* 242-250.

Paone, D., Cooper, H., Alperen, J., Shi, Q., & Des Jarlais, D. C. (1999). HIV risk behaviors of current sex workers attending syringe exchange: The experiences of women in five US cities. *AIDS Care, 11,* 269-280.

Pyett, P. M., & Warr, D. J. (1997). Vulnerability on the streets: Female sex workers and HIV risk. *AIDS Care, 9,* 539-547.

Reif, S., Wechsberg, W. M., & Dennis, M. L. (2001). Reduction of co-occurring distress in HIV risk behaviors among women substance abusers. *Journal of Prevention & Intervention in the Community, 22*(2), 61-80.

Rhodes, T., & Donoghoe, M. (1994). HIV prevalence no higher among female drug injectors also involved in prostitution. *AIDS Care, 6*(269-276).

Romans, S. E., Potter, K., Martin, J., & Herbison, P. (2001). The mental and physical health of female sex workers: A comparative study. *Australian and New Zealand Journal of Psychiatry, 35,* 75-80.

Silbert, M. H., & Pines, A. M. (1983). Early sexual exploitation as an influence in prostitution. *Social Work, 28,* 285-289.

Spittal, P. M., Bruneau, J., Craib, K. J. P., Miller, C., Lamothe, F., Weber, A. E., Li, K., Tyndall, M. W., O'Shaughnessy, M. V., & Schechter, M. T. (2003). Surviving the sex trade: A comparison of HIV risk behaviors among street-involved women in two Canadian cities who inject drugs. *AIDS Care, 15*(2), 187-195.

Stiffman, A. R., Doré, P., Felton, E., & Cunningham, R. (1992). The influence of mental health problems on AIDS-related risk behaviors in young adults. *The Journal of Nervous and Mental Disease, 180*(5), 314-320.

Surratt, H. L., Inciardi, J. A., Kurtz, S. P., & Kiley, M. C. (2004). Sex work and drug use in a subculture of violence. *Crime & Delinquency, 50*(1), 43-59.

Teets, J. M. (1995). Childhood sexual trauma of chemically dependent women. *Journal of Psychoactive Drugs, 27*(3), 231-238.

UNAIDS. (2004). *2004 report on the global AIDS epidemic: 4th global report.* Geneva, Switzerland: Author.

Valera, R. J., Sawyer, R. G., & Schiraldi, G. R. (2001). Perceived health needs of inner-city street prostitutes: A preliminary study. *American Journal of Health Behavior, 25*(1), 50-59.

Waldorf, D. (1973). *Careers in dope.* Englewood Cliffs, NJ: Prentice-Hall, Inc.

Watters, J. K., & Biernacki, P. (1989). Targeted sampling: Options for the study of hidden populations. *Social Problems, 36*(4), 416-430.

Weatherby, N., Needle, R. H., Cesari, H., Booth, R., McCoy, C., Watters, J., Williams, M., & Chitwood, D. (1994). Validity of self-reported drug use among injection drug users and crack cocaine users recruited through street outreach. *Evaluation and Program Planning, 17,* 347-355.

Wechsberg, W. M., Lam, W. K. K., Zule, W., Hall, G., Middlesteadt, R., & Edwards, J. (2003). Violence, homelessness, and HIV risk among crack-using African-American women. *Substance Use and Misuse, 38,* 669-700.

Wechsberg, W. M., MacDonald, B., Inciardi, J. A., Surratt, H. L., Leukefeld, C. G., Farabee, D., Cottler, L. B., Compton, W., Hoffman, J., Desmond, D., & Zule, W. (1997). *The NIDA cooperative agreement standard intervention: Protocol changes suggested by the continuing HIV/AIDS epidemic.* Bloomington, IL: Lighthouse Institute Publications.

Weiner, A. (1996). Understanding the social needs of streetwalking prostitutes. *Social Work, 41*(1), 97-105.

Wenzel, S. L., Leake, B. D., & Gelberg, L. (2001). Risk factors for major violence among homeless women. *Journal of Interpersonal Violence, 16*(8), 739-752.

Widom, C. S., & Ames, M. A. (1994). Criminal consequences of childhood sexual victimization. *Child Abuse and Neglect, 18*(4), 303-318.

Widom, C. S., Weiler, B. L., & Cottler, L. B. (1999). Childhood victimization and drug abuse: A comparison of prospective and retrospective findings. *Journal of Consulting and Clinical Psychology, 67*(6), 867-880.

Wiebel, W. W. (1990). Identifying and gaining access to hidden populations. In Lambert E. Y. (Ed.), *NIDA Research Monograph: The collection and interpretation of data from hidden populations* (Vol. 98, pp. 4-11). Rockville, MD: National Institute on Drug Abuse.

Wiebel, W. W. (1993). *The indigenous leader outreach model, NIH Publication No. 93-3581.* Rockville, MD: U.S. Department of Health and Human Services.

Williams, T. (1992). *Crackhouse: Notes from the end of the line.* Reading, MA: Addison-Wesley Publishing Company, Inc.

Wilsnack, S. C., Vogeltanz, N. D., Klassen, A. D., & Harris, T. R. (1997). Childhood sexual abuse and women's substance abuse: National survey findings. *Journal of Studies on Alcohol, May,* 264-271.

Young, A. M., Boyd, C., & Hubbell, A. (2000). Prostitution, drug use, and coping with psychological distress. *Journal of Drug Issues, 30*(4), 789-800.

Impact of Social and Structural Influence Interventions on Condom Use and Sexually Transmitted Infections Among Establishment-Based Female Bar Workers in the Philippines

Donald E. Morisky, ScD, ScM, MSPH
Chi Chiao, MSc, MSPH
Judith A. Stein, PhD
Robert Malow, PhD

Donald E. Morisky, Chi Chiao and Judith A. Stein are affiliated with the University of California, Los Angeles, CA.

Robert Malow is affiliated with the Florida International University, Miami, FL.

Address correspondence to: Donald E. Morisky, ScD, MSPH, ScM, University of California, Los Angeles, School of Public Health, 650 Charles E. Young Drive South, Los Angeles, CA 90095-1772 (E-mail: dmorisky@ucla.edu).

This research was supported by grant R01-AI33845 from the National Institutes of Allergy and Infectious Diseases to Donald E. Morisky, and grant PO1-DA-01070-30 to Judith A. Stein from the National Institute on Drug Abuse. The authors would like to thank Co-Investigator Teodora Tiglao, Research Managers Daisy Mejilla and Charlie Mendoza, and Site Coordinators Dorcas Romen, Mildred Publico, Angie Casas, and Lolipil Gella.

[Haworth co-indexing entry note]: "Impact of Social and Structural Influence Interventions on Condom Use and Sexually Transmitted Infections Among Establishment-Based Female Bar Workers in the Philippines." Morisky, Donald E. et al. Co-published simultaneously in *Journal of Psychology & Human Sexuality* (The Haworth Press, Inc.) Vol. 17, No. 1/2, 2005, pp. 45-63; and: *Contemporary Research on Sex Work* (ed: Jeffrey T. Parsons) The Haworth Press, Inc., 2005, pp. 45-63. Single or multiple copies of this article are available for a fee from The Haworth Document Delivery Service [1-800-HAWORTH, 9:00 a.m. - 5:00 p.m. (EST). E-mail address: docdelivery@haworthpress.com].

SUMMARY. This quasi-experimental study evaluated the influence of structural intervention components (e.g., changing organizational and social influence factors) in reducing biological sexually transmitted infections (STIs) and reports of unprotected sex among female bar workers (FBWs) in the Philippines (N = 369 at baseline). Recruited from four large southern Philippines cities, FBWs were exposed to a standard care, a manager influence, a peer influence, or a combined manager/peer influence condition. After the two-year intervention period, FBWs in the combined peer and manager intervention condition showed greater reductions in STIs and unprotected sex relative to those in the standard care condition. FBWs in the combined and the manager only conditions also showed a decrease in STIs compared to those in the standard care condition. Managers in the standard care condition reported lower positive condom attitudes and lower attendance at HIV/AIDS related training sessions compared to those in the combined condition. The combined effect of managers and peers had a positive, synergistic effect on condom use behavior and STI reduction compared to the standard care. This research provides empirical evidence that structural changes such as rules, regulations, and increased accessibility of condoms must be in combination with normative changes (individuals' attitudes, beliefs and normative expectancies) in order to achieve the greatest benefit in condom use behavior and STI reduction/prevention. *[Article copies available for a fee from The Haworth Document Delivery Service: 1-800-HAWORTH. E-mail address: <docdelivery@haworthpress.com> Website: <http://www.HaworthPress.com> © 2005 by The Haworth Press, Inc. All rights reserved.]*

KEYWORDS. Female bar workers, HIV/AIDS risk, structural intervention, STIs, condom use

In the Asian sex industry, commercial sex related activity has been transitioning outside of the brothel as legal pressures escalate and as customers perceive this pressure. Thus, increasing proportions of female sex workers are now operating in such venues as beer gardens, bars, nightclubs, karaoke TV centers, massage parlors, or disco dance establishments (Hanenberg & Rojanapithayakorn, 1998; WHO, 2001), where they have become known as indirect sex workers or as female bar workers (FBWs).

The FBWs' lifestyle tends to be particularly distinctive from that of brothel based sex workers who are commonly referred to as commercial sex workers (CSWs). This is especially true in the realm of heterosexual relationships (Bloom et al., 2002). Unlike brothel-based CSWs, FBWs predominantly host or entertain male customers within the confines of the establishment by serving drinks, conversing or other similar activities. FBWs receive only small salaries and/or commissions based on quantity of drinks and food items which they serve. FBWs generally negotiate sexual activities inside the work establishment, which typically take place off-premise. If the negotiated off-premise activities do occur during "working hours," the patron is generally expected to pay a "bar fine" to the establishment's manager for any of the FBWs "leave-time."

The FBWs' compensation for this negotiated off-premise sex work tends to be much greater than the meager establishment wages and is perceived as necessary to support basic individual and family survival needs. Unfortunately, these negotiated outside sexual activities often expose FBWs to a extraordinary risk of STI/HIV as well as other dangers within unseemly, unsupervised and coercive environments in which the power and financial dynamics are unsupportive of safe sex activities. This is likely to contribute to the epidemic spread of STIs, particularly HIV through the direct effects of these activities and through acquiring ulcerative STI which facilitates HIV transmission (Davis & Weller, 1999; WHO, 2002). Indeed, recent surveillance data documents a markedly higher level of STI/HIV seroprevalence among FBWs relative to the general population. For instance, in Thailand HIV seroprevalence among FBWs averages six times higher than in the general female adult population (WHO, 2001).

Since the initial AIDS case was reported in 1984 in the Philippines, the country has witnessed relatively low rates of HIV, and continues to be classified as a "low level" area (UNAIDS, 2001). The Joint United Nations Program on HIV/AIDS reported that approximately 10,000 individuals were living with HIV/AIDS in the Philippines at the end of 2001, yielding an adult infection rate of approximately .06 percent. Heterosexual transmission accounted for almost two-thirds of cases, followed by sex between men and bisexual contact. Less than .5 percent of transmissions occurred through injecting drug use (UNAIDS, 2001).

For 10 major Philippine cities, sentinel surveillance was undertaken to assess HIV/AIDS seroprevalence among registered female sex workers (RFSW), freelance female sex workers (FLSW), men who have sex with men (MSM), and injecting drug users. However, due to relatively minute seroprevalence of IDUs, a sufficiently sized sample was not obtainable, despite using all sentinel sites. The primary findings indicated that infection rates remained minuscule (< 1%), even among high-risk groups with the greatest prevalence among RFSW, who showed an aggregate prevalence rate ranging from 0.07% to 0.2% collectively for all sites (WHO, 1999).

Several underlying dynamics have maintained a relatively low STI/HIV prevalence in the Philippines. According to a United Nations Development Program report (WHO, 2002), favorable factors include: (1) circumcision which reduces transmission; (2) a lack of land borders combined with many islands that discourage intermixing; (3) a sexually conservative culture; (4) the most popular illicit drugs (e.g., marijuana and methamphetamine) are not injected so HIV transmission through sharing injection equipment is reduced; (5) national, multisector policies conducive toward reducing HIV/AIDS; (6) effective educational and information dissemination campaigns; and (7) comparative low numbers of sex partners among RFSW (2.5 per week in the Philippines vs. 4.5 per day in Thailand) (Morisky et al., 1998).

Commercial sex workers (CSWs), including those operating in brothel as well as non-traditional settings (e.g., bars, nightclubs, beer gardens) remain a priority group for STI/HIV prevention. Consistent with common beliefs, accumulating data support the contention that CSWs are contributing to the spread of HIV to heterosexuals (Reed, Ford, & Wirawan, 2001). As such, a burgeoning literature in this area has emerged regarding risk and protective factors for STI/HIV transmission (Sugihantono et al., 2003).

Established individual-level informational and attitudinal correlates of high risk behavior have been the focus of HIV prevention interventions. However, economic, organizational, legal and other macro-level structural factors have been increasingly emphasized in preventing HIV (Liu & So, 1996; Sumartojo, 2000). For example, reductions in HIV risk implemented by CSWs have been attributed to social-structural and external environmental determinants, such as workplace availability of condoms (Fontanet et al., 1998), policies mandating condom use between CSW and clients (Sedyaningsih Mamahit, 1996), HIV education programs (Ford et al., 1996), and the support of establishment owners and managers (Morisky et al., 1998; 2002).

The emerging literature on macro-level structural factors has prompted studies such as the present one which seeks to examine various non-brothel settings (see above) where commercial sex is negotiated. Because this area of research is neglected, the aim is to develop a better understanding of commercial sex exchange in non-brothel settings to guide the design of more tailored interventions to specifically reduce risk in this context.

The interventions used in this community longitudinal study are based on a combination of two theoretical frameworks, social cognitive theory at the individual level and social influence theory at the organizational level. STI prevention requires individuals to exercise influence over their own behaviors and their social environment. To achieve self-directed change, individuals need to be equipped not only with heightened awareness and knowledge but also with the behavioral means, resources and social support. Bandura (1986) has conceptualized the basic ingredients of social cognitive theory to consist of personal determinants in the form of cognitive, affective, biological factors, behavior, and the environment. This theoretical framework was applied to HIV/AIDS-related behaviors by not only teaching safer sex guidelines, but also equipping individuals with skills and self-beliefs that enable them to put the guidelines consistently into practice in the face of counteracting influences (Bandura, 1994).

The second theoretical framework used in this research consists of power and social influence. The social psychological study of power and influence finds its origin in the groundbreaking work of Kurt Lewin (1941). He considered power the possibility of inducing force on someone else, or, more formally, as the maximum force person A can induce on person B divided by the maximum resistance that B can offer. This conceptualization of power and social influence was further developed by French and Raven (1959), who defined influence as a force one person (the agent) exerts on someone else (the target) to induce a change in the target, including changes in behaviors, opinions, attitudes, goals, needs, and values. Social power was subsequently defined as the potential ability of an agent to influence a target. Raven further classified the six bases of power to include reward, coercive, legitimate, referent, expert and informational power (Raven, 1965). In a recent study, women who perceived that they have more power or share power reported significantly higher rates of condom use compared to those who perceived that their partners have more power (Harvey et al., 2002).

METHODS

Interventions

Four large cities (pop. > 200,000) located approximately 250 miles south of the Philippine capital (Manila) were identified as potential intervention sites. All organizations unanimously agreed to participate in the longitudinal study and were informed that they could have been assigned to an intervention group or a standard control group. Human subject approval was obtained from the Institutional Review Board of each participating university (UCLA and the University of the Philippines). The four participating sites were randomly assigned to one of the three intervention groups (peer counseling, manager training, or the combination of peer counseling and manager training) or to a standard control group.

The peer counseling intervention was implemented in all participating establishments in Site 1. In consultation with the manager/owner, two FBW from each establishment were selected and trained during a 5-day period at a nearby location. Travel allowances and a daily stipend were provided to defray expenses and lost work time. Content areas of the training program included basic information on STI and HIV, modes of transmission, interpersonal relationships with peers and clients in the work establishment, sexual negotiation, role playing and modeling, and normative expectancies. The manager training intervention in Site 2 consisted of the same topics as the peer counselors with additional training on their social influence role as a manager/supervisor by providing positive reinforcement of their employees' healthy sexual practices. Managers were encouraged to implement a continuum of educational policies, beginning with current practices, and gradually increasing to greater levels of involvement. These policies consisted of meeting regularly with their employees, monitoring their attendance at the SHC, providing educational materials on HIV/AIDS prevention, reinforcing positive STI prevention behaviors, attending monthly managers' advisory committee meetings, promoting AIDS awareness in the establishments (through posters, pamphlets, and brochures), providing educational materials to customers, making condoms available to FBW as well as to customers, and having a 100% condom use policy (oral and written). The combined intervention of peer counselors and manager training was implemented in two contiguous cities located in Site 3. Site 4, the standard control group, continued to receive standard treatment which consisted of regular examinations at the Social Hygiene Clinic (SHC). All sites are geographically dispersed throughout the southern Philippines, resulting in minimal potential for contamination.

Participants and Procedures

Four non-contiguous locations in the southern Philippines (southern Luzon, Cebu, Ilo-Ilo and northern Mindanao) were selected owing to few ongoing HIV/AIDS prevention programs. Participants were informed of the objectives of the study and the potential risks and benefits of participation. All of the individuals who agreed to participate in the research (greater than 98%) completed an informed consent form. The participants were selected on a voluntary basis and were recruited from all entertainment-related establishments in which FBWs were employed (e.g., bars, nightclubs, beer gardens, karaoke bar, massage parlor, and hotels). Through face-to-face interviews, 1383 CSWs were interviewed from 105 establishments, including 936 bar-based workers along with their employers at the time of the baseline assessment. At the time of the post-test assessment, responses were obtained from 1484 CSWs from 145 establishments, including 986 bar-based workers and their employers. In this current study, we focus on the subgroup of FBWs who reported having received payment for sexual relations with customers during a one month period prior to the survey and especially employed at bars, nightclubs, beer gardens, discos, and karaoke bars. From the baseline survey the sample included 369 FBWs from 60 establishments (15 in Legaspi, 19 in Cagayan, 19 in Cebu, and 7 in Ilo-Ilo). From post-test interviews the sample included 371 FBWs from 75 establishments (13 in Legaspi, 21 in Cagayan, 30 in Cebu, and 11 in Ilo-Ilo). The repeated measure, cross sectional study did not necessarily have the same women participating in the baseline and post-test samples. FBWs' perception of the attitudes and beliefs of their establishment's managers were obtained at pre- and post-test assessment from 60 and 75 managers respectively.

Measures

The present research is part of a large-scale community survey using a participatory research approach. The study included two primary components: (1) a baseline and post-intervention survey 2 years interval for both FBWs and managers in the respective establishments; (2) a prospective assessment of STI rates among FBWs. The survey consisted of 134 items. Personal interviews were conducted in the native dialect with FBWs and their establishment managers, supervisors or owners in the establishments in which they are employed. All instruments were back translated into English, with over 98% agreement among FBWs and 100% among managers/supervisors.

The FBW survey covered demographics, knowledge, attitudes, beliefs, risk behavior, perception of own risk for HIV infection, self-efficacy for condom use, alcohol and drug use and social desirability. The survey instrument developed for managers also measured attitudes and beliefs as related to perceptions of risk-taking behaviors by employees and customers and the level of support provided to employees for condom use. The manager survey also assessed characteristics of the work environment that reinforce less risky sexual behaviors such as the provision of AIDS prevention classes or educational materials for workers; the existence of mandatory condom use policy; condom provision.

The measures used in this current study included reports from the FBWs about establishment practice, manager attitudes, manager training, condom use behaviors and biologically validated STI results from the SHC. Establishment practices were operationalized by three items addressing rules and communications operating within the establishment. These items included: (1) Whether a co-worker at her establishment had ever tried to convince her to use a condom with a customer; (2) whether her establishment has a rule that all workers must use condoms when having sex with customers; and (3) whether her boss ever talked to her about using condoms. All measures were dichotomous responses (yes/no). Four items (assessed from managers) represent their attitudes based on scaled statements about condoms ranging from strongly agree (1) to strongly disagree (5). These items included: (1) A bar would lose many customers, if it requires workers to use condoms; (2) the manager should require workers to use condoms, even though it is against their religion; (3) it is the customers' decision to use condoms; (4) it is bad for business to talk about AIDS prevention. Finally, three items obtained from the manager were used to quantify their AIDS training activities. These items addressed whether or not the manager attended an AIDS training/education class, participated in monthly community meeting with other managers, and whether or not the manager attended a condom use class.

Two major outcome indicators were condom use behavior and STI. The first indicator was assessed by a validated six-item scale, having an alpha reliability coefficient of .80 (Morisky, Ang, and Sneed, 2002). These items included scaled questions ranging from 1 (never) to 5 (always) that include examples of questions that ask how often FBWs "use a condom when engaging in vaginal sex," "suggest using a condom to their partner," "carry a condom on their person." A summated score was calculated after reversed-coded adjustment. The likelihood of using condoms was estimated by total scores divided by the maximum scores (30). The second indicator was whether the FBWs had been diagnosed with an STI in the past month. This variable was coded as yes (1) and no (0). This measure was based on the results of a clinic chart review of all visits to the SHC during the month preceding the survey. The ratio of the number of SHC visits made during the month preceding the survey divided by the number of weeks the FBW was working in the establishment during this same period (Person Weeks) is used to assess potential STI selection biases.

Data Analysis

All analyses were performed with SPSS-PC version 10.0. Bivariate analyses with Chi-square tests for categorical variables were used to determine the statistical significance of all comparisons (individual socio-demographics and social influence impacts) among FBWs from four study groups. Chi-square tests were used to assess differentials concerning establishment practices and policies, attitudes towards condom use and enforcing a condom-use policy, and attendance at AIDS training programs in the community and STI. Analysis of variance was used to assess the relative effects of the different interventions on condom use behavior, followed by regression models, controlling for hypothesized confounding factors.

RESULTS

Background of FBWs

Table 1 presents data on social and demographic characteristics of study populations from the baseline interview and post-test assessment. At baseline the 369 FBWs employed at bar/club/beer garden (63%), discos (28%), and karaoke bar (9%) were included in analyses. The ages of these FBWs ranged from 15-39 years (m = 22.4) and they averaged 8.5 years of school. Their average work duration was 11.20 months. Ten percent of the FBWs were married and 53.8% reported having at least one child. Average weekly income was 1166.5 pesos (approximately $50 US). In the post-test assessment, analyses included 371 FBWs working at bars/clubs/beer gardens (45%), discos (14%), and karaoke bars (42%). Participants ranged in age from 15-41 years (m = 22.3), worked an average of 11.3 months, and had an average of 8.3 years of education. Only 8% of the population was married, with 55.3% of participants reporting having at least one child. Average weekly income was 1372.5 pesos or approximately $50/week, based on a devaluation of the Philippine peso between the two time intervals.

TABLE 1. Distribution (Mean [Std Dev]/Numbers [Percentage]) of Socio-Demographic Characteristics of the FBW Participants by Study Groups at Baseline and Post-Test Assessments

	Peer Education (Legaspi)		Manager Training (Cagayan)		Combined Intervention (Cebu)		Standard Care (Ilo-Ilo)		Total		Statistic test	
	Pre (n = 80)	Post (n = 33)	Pre (n = 132)	Post (n = 57)	Pre (n = 115)	Post (n = 219)	Pre (n = 42)	Post (n = 62)	Pre (n = 369)	Post (n = 370)	Pre	Post
Mean age in years	24.29 (4.80)	23.03 (6.28)	22.27 (3.95)	23.75 (4.27)	22.06 (3.81)	22.02 (4.24)	20.07 (2.03)	21.42 (3.41)	22.39 (4.11)	22.27 (3.41)	$F_{3,365} = 11.31$***	$F_{3,367} = 3.60$*
Mean schooling in years	8.26 (1.95)	7.85 (2.05)	8.77 (1.82)	7.93 (2.37)	8.08 (2.06)	8.32[c] (2.03)[b]	9.29 (1.42)	8.56 (2.06)	8.50 (1.92)	8.26 (2.10)	$F_{3,365} = 5.36$*	$F_{3,366} = 1.39$
Work duration in months	8.23 (7.75)	10.30 (8.40)	13.20 (15.73)	12.95 (10.37)	8.65 (9.28)	9.07 (11.15)	8.79 (9.07)	18.13 (17.92)	10.20 (11.91)	11.29 (12.64)	$F_{3,365} = 4.49$*	$F_{3,367} = 9.28$***
Mean weekly wage in pesos	793.04 (599.61)	1460.67 (1331.36)	1087.73 (776.51)	921.58 (542.68)	1137.30 (903.13)	1400.94 (1067.79)	2221.95 (2011.41)	1639.52 (1419.11)	1166.54 (1070.54)	1372.47 (1116.29)	$F_{3,365} = 19.26$***	$F_{3,367} = 4.52$*
Marital status[a] Living alone	53 (66.30%)	22[c] (68.80%)	86 (65.20%)	37 (64.90%)	94 (81.70%)	167[d] (76.60%)	31 (73.80%)	31 (50.00%)	264 (71.50%)	257 (69.60%)	$X^2 = 9.73$* df = 3	$X^2 = 16.93$* df = 3
Married or single living with boyfriend	27 (33.80%)	10[c] (31.30%)	46 (34.80%)	20 (35.10%)	21 (18.30%)	51[c] (23.40%)	11 (26.20%)	31 (50.00%)	105 (28.50%)	112 (30.40%)		
Recruitment into sex work[b] by advertisement	31 (38.80%)	16 (48.50%)	82 (62.1%)	40 (70.20%)	48 (41.70%)	73 (33.30%)	17[e] (43.60%)	12 (19.40%)	178 (48.60%)	141 (38.00%)	$X^2 = 15.33$* df = 3	$X^2 = 37.76$*** df = 3
self/other	49 (61.30%)	17 (51.50%)	50 (37.90%)	17 (29.80%)	67 (58.30%)	146 (66.70%)	22[e] (56.40%)	50 (80.60%)	188 (51.40%)	230 (62.00%)		

[a] Marital status: FBWs categorized as living alone include single (never married), separated (living alone), and widowed. For those who were categorized as living with somebody else, they were single but living with their boyfriend and married (s/b).

[b] Recruitment was categorized into 2 levels. One was recruited by answering an ad or applied by self. Another was recruited by other venues, including a friend, relative, or family member, a mamasan, an establishment owner, or employment agency.

[c] One case in Cebu did not respond to question regarding her schooling at the post-test assessment.

[d] There was one case in Legaspi and one case in Cebu, who did not respond to the question regarding marital status at post-test assessment.

[e] Three cases in Ilo-Ilo site did not respond to the question regarding recruitments into sex work at the baseline assessment.

*** refers to p-value < .0001   ** refers to p-value < .001   * refers to p-value < .05.

54

Comparisons of the FBWs from the baseline and those from post-test assessments indicate similar social and demographic characteristics, except for weekly income. The FBWs from the post-test assessment had higher incomes than the FBWs from the baseline interviews. However, there is significant variation across the four sites for most social and demographic characteristics at the baseline and post-test assessments.

Social Influence

Table 2 presents the relationship between social influence (establishment practice, manager attitude, and manager training) and the four study sites post intervention. A higher proportion of positive establishment practice concerning condom use behavior was found in the combination intervention site at post-test assessment. Almost all FBWs in this site reported their establishments had a rule (99%) and reported that their boss talked to them about using condoms (98%); in contrast to the standard care study site in Ilo-Ilo (82%; $\chi^2_{(3)} = 86.59$, p < .001; 65%; $\chi^2_{(3)} = 79.59$, p < .001, respectively).

Manager attitudes concerning condom use behaviors were significantly more positive in the combination site compared to other sites. For example, while none of the managers in the combination site agreed or strongly agreed that a bar would lose many customers if it required workers to use condoms, 53% in the control site agreed. Furthermore, only 12% of the managers in the combined intervention site stated that it is the customers' decision to use condoms; 42% in the standard treatment site agreed. Managers from the combined intervention group were also less likely to agree or strongly agree that talking about AIDS prevention was bad for business, whereas 10% in the peer education site, 35% in manager site, and 52% in the control site agreed or strongly agreed ($\chi^2_{(3)} = 130.21$, p < .001). Finally, all managers in the combination site agreed or strongly agreed that their workers should be required to use condoms even though it may be against their religion; in contrast to 76% in the manager training site and 57% in the standard care site ($\chi^2_{(3)} = 107.27$, p < .001).

The managers in the combined intervention site were also significantly more likely to participate in training programs addressing HIV/AIDS prevention compared to managers in other sites. Approximately 91% of the managers in the combined intervention site, for instance, attended AIDS education classes, compared to 87% in the peer education site, 48% in the manager training site, and 58% in the stan-

TABLE 2. Frequencies of Establishment Practice, Manager Attitude and Manager Training by Study Group at the Post-Test Assessment (n = 371)

	Peer Education (Legaspi)	Manager Training (Cagayan)	Combined Intervention (Cebu)	Standard Treatment (Ilo-Ilo)	$x^2_{(3)}$
Establishment practice					
1. Your co-workers try to convince you to use a condom with a customer.	68.80%	54.40%	58.70%	75.80%	8.01*
2. Your establishment has a rule that all workers must use condoms when having sex with customers.	86.70%	53.70%	98.60%	82.30%	86.59***
3. Your boss ever talked to you about using condoms.	73.30%	59.30%	98.20%	64.50%	79.59***
Manager attitudes					
If you strongly agree or agree: 1. A bar would lose many customers, if it requires workers to use condoms	0.00%	22.00%	0.00%	53.20%	128.71[a]***
2. The manager should require workers to use condoms, even though it is against their religion.	100.00%	75.90%	100.00%	56.50%	107.27***
3. It is customers' decision to use condoms.	46.70%	46.30%	12.40%	41.90%	48.19***
4. It is bad for business to talk about AIDS prevention.	10.00%	35.20%	0.00%	51.60%	130.21[a]***
Manager training					
You attended:					
1. AIDS education classes.	86.70%	48.10%	91.30%	58.10%	67.89***
2. Community meetings about AIDS.	70.00%	57.40%	86.70%	66.10%	28.62***
3. Condom use classes in the past 6 months.	73.30%	70.40%	75.20%	61.30%	4.75

[a]Likelihood ratio is used, instead of Pearson's Chi Square, since there is at least one cell that has expected count less than 5.
* p < .05; ** p < .001; *** p < .0001

dard care site ($\chi^2_{(3)} = 67.89$, p < .001). In the combined intervention site, establishment managers were more likely to participate in community meetings about AIDS (87%) compared to managers in the peer education site (70%), the manager training site (57%), and the standard treatment site (66%) ($\chi^2_{(3)} = 28.62$, p < .001).

Condom Use Behavior

The combined intervention site had the highest reported likelihood of consistent condom use behavior among FBWs (93%); in contrast to 80% in the peer education site, 73% in the manager training site, and 58% in the standard treatment site (F = 128.5, *df.* = 3, p < .001). Table 3 presents the results for condom use behaviors of FBWs across four study sites at pre- and post-test. Models 1 and 3 measure variations in condom use behaviors by study groups at pre- and post-test, respectively, by using simple regression models. Models 2 and 4 adjust for confounding factors such as age, education, work duration and weekly wage on condom use behavior among the four study sites. In the four models, the condom use scale is measured by a composite score comprised of six variables with a range of 6 to 30, and the standard treatment site 4 is selected as the reference group. In Model 1 FBWs assigned to the peer education group and the combined intervention group reported higher means of condom use compared to the standard treatment group at pre-test assessment by 11% (p < .05) and 16% (p < .0001), respectively. After adjusting for individual characteristics, Model 2 continued to demonstrate higher means of condom use.

Model 3 displays the crude intervention effects at post-test assessment and finds that FBWs in the combined group reported approximately 60% higher mean condom use scores compared to the standard

TABLE 3. Regressions of Condom Use Behavior on Intervention Effects Controlling for Individual Sociodemographic Characteristics [Unstandardized Coefficients (Std Dev)] from Baseline Interview and Post-Test Assessment

	Baseline (n = 369)		Post-test (n = 370)	
	Model 1 b (SE)	Model 2 b (SE)	Model 3 b (SE)	Model 4 b (SE)
Intervention effect				
Peer Education (Legaspi)[a]	2.34(1.05)*	4.14(1.16)***	6.40(0.89)***	6.45(0.92)***
Manager Training (Cagayan)[a]	0.47(0.86)	1.37(0.95)	4.33(0.75)***	4.68(0.79)***
Combined Intervention (Cebu)[a]	3.40(0.86)***	4.40(0.94)***	10.48(0.58)***	10.57(0.61)***
Individual Sociodemographic Characteristics				
Age		−0.20(0.07)*		−0.12(0.05)*
Education		0.56(0.14)***		0.11(0.10)
Work Duration		−0.01(0.02)		−0.00(0.02)
Weekly Wage		0.00(0.00)		−0.00(0.00)
Marital Status (ref = living alone) Living with sb		−0.22(0.58)		0.03(0.47)
Recruitment to work (ref = AD or self) Recruited by others		0.16(0.53)		−0.52(0.43)
INTERCEPT	20.91(0.74)***	19.70(2.17)***	17.52(0.53)***	18.91(1.43)***
R²	0.11	0.20	0.54	0.56

[a] Reference group = Standard Care Group at Ilo-Ilo Site
* p < .05; ** p < .001; *** p < .0001

care group (p < .0001), followed by FBWs at the peer counseling site (37%; p < .0001) and the manager training groups (25%; p < .0001). After adjusting for individual sociodemographic characteristics in Model 4, the intervention effects remain significant compared to the standard care group.

In contrast to the standard care group, the predicted mean changes in condom use between pre- and post-test assessment were found across all three intervention groups when considering individual socioeconomic characteristics. The most significant change was found in the combined intervention group. A two sample t-test was conducted to assess pre-post differentials. As noted in Table 4, a means comparison of predicted values in condom use behavior demonstrated highly significant differences between pre- and post-test assessment, with a t-value of 30.73 (p < .0001) even after controlling for individual characteristics.

STI Status

In the post-test assessments, the combined intervention site (Cebu) had the lowest observed STI infection rate (27%) followed by 40% in the manager training site (Cagayan de Oro), 53% in the standard treatment site (Ilo-Ilo), and 67% in the peer education site (Legaspi City) ($\chi^2 = 29.3$, $df. = 3$, p < .001). Figure 1 indicates that STI rates were significantly lower for FBWs in the manager training and combined intervention groups compared to those in the other groups. While 27% of FBWs in the combined intervention site and 40% in the manager training site had

TABLE 4. Predicted Values of Condom Use Behavior Adjusted for Individual Sociodemographic Characteristics at Baseline and Post-Test Assessments [Means (Std Dev)]

	Peer Education (Site 1)	Manager Training (Site 2)	Combined (Site 3)	Standard Treatment (Site 4)
Baseline Assessment	23.25(1.17)	21.38(2.56)	24.31(1.42)	20.86(2.15)
Post-test Assessment	23.88(3.15)	21.85(1.93)	27.99(0.78)	17.52(1.13)
Change from Baseline to Post-test[a]	+0.63	+0.47	+3.68	−3.34
t-test[b]	$t_{111} = 2.63^*$	$t_{187} = 1.24^*$	$t_{332} = 30.73^{***}$	$t_{109} = -11.23^{***}$

[a]Positive sign means increase in condom use from baseline to follow-up assessment. Negative sign means decrease in condom use from baseline to follow-up assessment.
[b]Independent t-test. * p < .05; ** p < .001; *** p < .0001

FIGURE 1. STI Rate by Study Group at Post-Test (χ^2 = 29.3, *df.* = 3, p < .001)

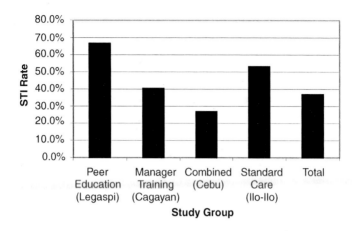

STI infection three months after intervention, 67% of FBWs in the peer ed-ucation group and 53% in the standard treatment group were found to have an STI (χ^2 = 29.3, *df.* = 3, p < .001).

DISCUSSION

This study is one of the first analyses of the effects of a quasi-experi-mental behaviorally oriented intervention hypothesized to affect the so-cial influence on condom use behavior and STI among a high-risk group of female bar workers who reported having received payment for sex. The interventions were directed at the individual level (social modeling factors) as well as the organizational level (social-structural and envi-ronment factors). Participants in the combined study site were found to benefit most from the structural interventions in terms of increased es-tablishment practices addressing educational policy, greater level of manager involvement, and more positive manager attitudes towards condom use behavior. The fact that a high proportion of managers in the standard treatment site (53%) indicated that the bar would lose many customers if they required customers to use condoms reflects the nega-tive attitudes and lack of positive reinforcement between managers and employees. Managers in the intervention sites were encouraged to become actively involved in the ongoing positive reinforcement of safe sexual practices among their employees. This included actively discussing negotiation and communication skills during weekly meetings, the importance of their employees' health and economic hardships for their family when considering non-condom use. FBWs were encouraged to discuss and negotiate sexual activities to take place after work hours in the establishment so they can avail of the positive support of their managers. Managers in turn were instructed to be supportive of safe sexual behaviors whenever customers would try to convince the FBW not to use condoms. This resulted in greater assurance on the part of the FBW that her manager would support her in safe sexual negotiations with potential clients.

It is interesting that consistent condom use behavior was found to rank second highest in the peer education site, however this did not translate into lower STI rates among the FBW. In fact, the STI rate was found to be highest in the peer education site. Further analysis into the proper use of condoms among FBWs in this intervention site was obtained by analyzing the question "during the past month, did you ever have a condom fall off inside you during sexual intercourse." Responses to this question revealed that the peer education site had the highest probability of condom use failure among intervention groups, with FBWs reporting a 24% failure rate compared to 13% in the manager training site, 14% in the combined intervention site, and 30% in the standard treatment site ($\chi^2 = 8.1$, $df. = 3$, p < .044).

Most importantly, the results of the condom use behavior scale indicated significantly higher levels of consistent use among intervention sites, particularly in the combined intervention site. There was also a significant improvement in condom use behavior from pre to post test among all intervention sites, using the standard treatment site as a reference. This significant change over time was maintained even when controlling for possible confounding variables, including age, education, work duration and weekly average salary.

Study Limitations

The use of self reports to measure sensitive outcome behavior, such as condom use, was a potential source of bias in this study. This measure may be subject to error through a social desirability bias. However, the measure was assessed for any social desirability bias and no significant differences were found between individuals who stated they use condoms always or very often compared to individuals reporting using condoms less frequently (Morisky et al., 2002). Individuals who reported high condom use behavior were also found to have lower incidence of STI. Further research is recommended on quantifying this behavior in order to provide more reliable and valid measures. Another potential bias is the possibility that preexisting and uncontrollable site differences may have contributed to some of the results. However, considerable care was taken to select representative and comparable communities in the southern Philippines and randomly assign intervention approaches to each community.

Implications for Practice

This study identifies several important structural factors existing in the work environment that influence the use of condoms for female bar workers that are employed in a variety of entertainment establishments in the Philippines. The results suggest a need for the development of comprehensive educational policies in each of these identified establishments. Particularly important is the relationship between establishment managers and their employees. Holding regular meetings with employees provides opportunities to reinforce the importance of regular attendance at the SHC and promotes STI/HIV awareness. Having a policy that all workers must use condoms and providing free condoms in the workplace are key factors that positively influence condom use among FBWs. The most important implication for public health practice is the highly significant synergistic effects of the combination of the manager training component and the peer education intervention. The results highlight the inability of the managers to influence new social norms without somehow witnessing the interaction of their employees with designated peers. Structural changes, consisting of rules, regulations and educational policy, must work in combination with normative changes (individual changes in knowledge, positive beliefs and attitudes, and normative expectancies). This combined approach results in a participatory collaboration on the part of establishment managers and employees, leading to higher rates of consistent condom use behavior and reduced incidence of STIs. Finally, the participatory exchange can be expanded by encouraging city and municipal governments to enforce existing ordinances requiring FBWs to be registered at the SHC.

These findings present important implications for research and program planning in this field. As the setting and dynamics within which commercial sex occur have changed over time, so too must the development of STI and HIV prevention methodology and interventions to reflect the changing needs and reality of the women affected.

REFERENCES

Bandura, A. (1986). *Social foundations of thought and action: A social cognitive theory*. Englewood Cliffs, NJ: Prentice-Hall.

Bandura, A. (1994). Social Cognitive Theory and Exercise of Control over HIV Infection. In R.J. DiClemente and J.L. Peterson (Eds.), Preventing AIDS: Theories and Methods of Behavioral Interventions (pp. 25-59). New York: Plenum Press.

Bloom, S.S., Urassa, M., Isingo, R., Ng'weshemi, J., Boerma, J.T. (2002). Community effects on the risk of HIV infection in rural Tanzania. *Sex Transm Infect*, 78(4): 261-6.

Davis, K.R., Susan, C. Weller. (1999). The effectiveness of condoms in reducing heterosexual transmission of HIV. *Family Planning Perspectives*, 31(6): 272-279.

Fontanet, A.L., Saba, J., Chandelying, V., Sakondhavat, C., Bhiraleus, P., Rugpao, S., Chongsomchai, C., Kiriwat, O., Tovanabutra, S., Dally, L., Lange, J.M., Rojanapithayakorn, W. (1998). Protection against sexually transmitted diseases by granting sex workers in Thailand the choice of using the male or female condom: results from a randomized controlled trial. *AIDS*, 12 (14): 1851-1859.

Ford, K., Wirawan, D.N., Fajans, P., Meliawan, P., MacDonald, K., and Thorpe, L. (1996). Behavioral interventions for reduction of sexually transmitted disease/HIV transmission among female commercial sex workers and clients in Bali, Indonesia. *AIDS*, 10, 213-245.

French, J. R. P., Jr., & Raven, B. H. (1959). The bases of social power. In D. Cartwright (Ed.), *Studies in social power* (pp. 150-167). Ann Arbor, MI: Institute for Social Research.

Hanenberg, R., Rojanapithayakorn, W. (1998). Changes in prostitution and the AIDS epidemic in Thailand. *AIDS Care*. 10: 69-79.

Harvey, S. M., Bird, S.T., Galavotti, C., Duncan, E.A.W., & Greenberg, D. (2002). Relationship, power, sexual decision making and condom use among women at risk for HIV/STDs. *Women & Health*, 36 (4): 69-84.

Lewin, K. (1941). *Analysis of the concepts whole, differentiation, and unity*. University of Iowa Studies in Child Welfare, 18, 226-261.

Liu, T.I., So, R. (1996). Knowledge, Attitude, and Preventive Practice Survey Regarding AIDS Comparing Registered to Freelance Commercial Sex Workers in Iloilo City, Philippines. *Southeast Asian J Tropical Med Public Health*, 27:696-702.

Morisky, D. E., Stein, J. A., Sneed, C. D., Tiglao, T. V., Liu, K., Detels, R., Tempongko, S. B., & Baltazar, J. C. (2002). Modeling personal and situational influences on condom use among establishment-based commercial sex workers in the Philippines. *AIDS & Behavior*, 6, 163-172.

Morisky, D. E., Tiglao, T.V., Sneed, C. D., Tempongko, S. B., Baltazar, J. C., Detels, R. and Stein, J. A. (1998). The effects of establishment practices, knowledge and attitudes on condom use among Filipina sex workers. *AIDS Care, 10*, 213-220.

Morisky, D. E., Ang, A., Sneed, C.D. (2002). Validating the effects of social desirability on self-reported condom use behavior among commercial sex workers. *AIDS Education and Prevention*, 14(5): 351-60.

The Philippines Health Department. (1996). Technical report.

Raven, B. H. (1965). Social influence and power. In I. D. Steiner & M. Fishbein (Eds.), Current studies in social psychology (pp. 399-444). New York: Wiley.

Reed, B.D., Ford, K., Wirawan, D.N. (2001). The Bali STD/AIDS study: association between vaginal hygiene practices and STDs among sex workers. *Sex Transm Infect*, (1): 46-52.

Sedyaningsih-Mamahit, E.R. (1996). Clients and brothel managers in Kramat Tunggak, Jakarta, Indonesia: Interweaving qualitative with quantitative studies for planning STD/AIDS prevention programs. *Southeast Asian J Tropical Med Public Health* 28:513-524.

Sugihantono, A., Slidell, M., Syaifudin, A., Pratjojo, H., Utami, I.M., Sadjimin, T., Mayer, K.H. (2003). Syphilis and HIV prevalence among commercial sex workers in Central Java, Indonesia: Risk-taking behavior and attitudes that may potentiate a wider epidemic. *AIDS Patient Care and STDs*, 17 (11): 595-600.

Sumartojo, E. (2000). Structural factors in HIV prevention: concepts, examples, and implications for research. *AIDS* 14: S3-S10.

WHO (2002). http://www.who.int/hiv/pub/sti/en/who_hiv_2002_14.pdf

WHO (2001). http://www.wpro.who.int/pdf/sti/aids2001/part2_grp1.pdf

WHO (2001). Sex Work in Asia. (*http://www.wpro.who.int/document/FINAL-Sex% 20Work%20in%20Asia.doc*).

UNAIDS (2001). Country Profile: HIV/AIDS in the Philippines. (*http://www.synergyaids. com/documents/*Philippines_profile.pdf).

How Does a "Risk Group" Perceive Risk? Voices of Vietnamese Sex Workers in Cambodia

Joanna Busza, MSc

SUMMARY. Throughout the HIV/AIDS epidemic, female sex workers have been identified as a "risk group" and interventions developed to reduce their behavioral risk-taking. Both individual and structural level programs continue to target "risks" such as multiple partners and lack of condom use. Sex workers themselves, however, are likely to view their experiences more holistically, perceiving a range of risks within their work. This paper presents qualitative data from a participatory study conducted with brothel-based migrant Vietnamese sex workers in Cambodia, illuminating one community's perceptions of the sex industry. It argues that design and implementation of effective HIV prevention activities must be based on sex workers' own interpretations and responses to risk, using them as a realistic entry point for effecting change. Actively engaging with sex workers through participatory research and projects offers the first step in shifting the current epidemiological focus toward identifying feasible, context-specific risk-reduction strategies. *[Article copies available for a fee from The Haworth Document Delivery Service: 1-800-HAWORTH. E-mail address: <docdelivery@haworthpress.com> Website: <http://www.HaworthPress.com> © 2005 by The Haworth Press, Inc. All rights reserved.]*

Joanna Busza, MSc, is affiliated with the Centre for Population Studies, London School of Hygiene & Tropical Medicine, 49-51 Bedford Square, London WC1B 3DP, UK (E-mail: joanna.busza@lshtm.ac.uk).

[Haworth co-indexing entry note]: "How Does a 'Risk Group' Perceive Risk? Voices of Vietnamese Sex Workers in Cambodia." Busza, Joanna. Co-published simultaneously in *Journal of Psychology & Human Sexuality* (The Haworth Press, Inc.) Vol. 17, No. 1/2, 2005, pp. 65-82; and: *Contemporary Research on Sex Work* (ed: Jeffrey T. Parsons) The Haworth Press, Inc., 2005, pp. 65-82. Single or multiple copies of this article are available for a fee from The Haworth Document Delivery Service [1-800-HAWORTH, 9:00 a.m. - 5:00 p.m. (EST). E-mail address: docdelivery@haworthpress.com].

Digital Object Identifier: 10.1300/J056v17n01_05

KEYWORDS. Cambodia, brothels, sex work, HIV, risk

Throughout the HIV/AIDS epidemic, female sex workers have been identified as a "risk group" with higher rates of both susceptibility and transmission of the virus compared to the general population (UNAIDS, 2002a). As a result, research and interventions have targeted sex workers to study and change their behavioral risk profiles. Within this context, "risk-taking" generally refers to sex with multiple partners, lack of condom use, and, where relevant, injecting-drug use. Recently, the focus has shifted from individual to structural determinants of risk among sex workers, taking into consideration ways in which conditions in the sex industry shape sex workers' ability to negotiate safer practices (Parker, Easton & Klein, 2000). For the most part, investigations of "risk" have remained within an epidemiological framework and thus are limited to sexual behaviors, although advocates have called for more holistic perspectives in addressing sex workers' lives, including analysis of how sex workers themselves define "risk" (NSWP, 1997).

This paper presents qualitative data from an operations research study conducted among brothel-based migrant Vietnamese sex workers in Cambodia, illuminating one community's views of "risk-taking" in the sex industry. After a brief review of the literature, it offers sex workers' perspectives of how they identify and negotiate daily challenges. This case study suggests that "risk" embodies a range of concerns and priorities among sex workers that do not fit the public health paradigm, but require a wider analytical lens. HIV-prevention programs need to remain cognizant of pressures and motivations facing sex workers in order to develop feasible interventions to reduce their vulnerability to HIV. Actively engaging with sex workers through participatory research and projects can offer a first step in shifting risk-reduction strategies from an epidemiological approach to one better suited to developing feasible and context-specific means of social change.

From the earliest stages of the HIV pandemic, sex workers have attracted attention as a "risk group" because of their occupational exposure to multiple sexual partners and the key role that commercial sex has played in sustaining HIV transmission in some settings (UNAIDS, 1996). Most programs and policies aimed at sex workers have been based on an epidemiological understanding of HIV. This identified them as a "core group" with the potential to serve as a "reservoir of disease" and spread infections to the "general public" through the "bridging population" of clients (Day & Ward, 1997, Plummer et al., 1991).

Numerous surveys of sex workers' knowledge and behavior confirmed high levels of behavioral risk, particularly low condom use with clients (Joesoef et al., 2000, Lau, Tsui, Siah & Zhang, 2002, Wong et al., 2003).

In response, a range of public health measures have been put into place, encompassing various combinations of education, services and regulation, depending on the local legal and cultural context (Day & Ward, 1997). Commonly implemented measures include peer education programs, widespread distribution of male and female condoms, and increased access to "user-friendly" sexual and reproductive health services, including regular or presumptive treatment for sexually transmitted infections (STI) (Fontanet et al., 1998, Ford, Wirawan, Reed, Muliawan & Wolfe, 2002, Ray, van de Wijgert, Mason, Ndowa & Maposhere, 2001). On a larger scale, Thailand introduced a national "100% condom policy" that mandates condom use throughout the entire brothel-based sex sector. The success of this approach has led other countries, including Cambodia, to adopt it, albeit with some controversy (Hanenberg, Rojanapithayakorn, Kunasol & Sokal, 1994; Loff, Overs & Longo, 2003). These programs work within a public health framework and thus target behavior deemed "risky" by being implicated in spreading HIV to the general population.

In recent years, concern has grown for sex workers' own vulnerability to infection (Tawil et al., 1999, Wolffers & van Beelen, 2003). Reflecting a wider paradigm shift toward community mobilization in HIV prevention, attention has turned toward socio-cultural structures that shape the sex industry and thus the risks to which sex workers are exposed (Campbell, 2000, Parker et al., 2000). Research that has adopted this framework has highlighted sex workers' marginalised status within society, as well as their level of power vis-à-vis clients, managers, and law enforcement authorities (Campbell & Mzaidume, 2001, Pauw & Brener, 2003).

In this work, therefore, the extent of behavioral risk does not rely so much on individual sex workers' sexual health knowledge or motivation to use condoms but rather on the environment in which sex work occurs. Campbell (2000) and Wojcicki and Malala (2001) have demonstrated, for instance, how in South Africa, community-level constructs of predatory male sexuality and competition among women create conditions in which sex workers find it nearly impossible to control terms of trade or insist on condom use. Interventions based on such findings have worked to empower sex workers and contribute to the mobilization of their communities. These projects attempt to build self-esteem, critical thinking and peer support among sex workers in order to stimulate a context conducive to structural change. Perhaps most impressively, in Kolkata, India, the Sonagachi brothel district experienced a radical political awakening that not only increased condom use from 2.7% to 81.7%, maintaining HIV prevalence below 5%, but also launched a sustained sex workers' rights movement (Jana et al., 1998).

Yet programs based on community development for sex workers as a means to facilitate their ability to avoid sexual risk-taking have not all met with success. In Madras, a pilot empowerment project failed due to competition between sex workers and strict control of the sex industry by criminal networks (Asthana & Oostvogels, 1996). Similar barriers have been found in other settings (Campbell, 2003). In these cases, one factor inhibiting widespread behavioral change has been that numerous and wide-ranging "risks" such as loss of income or violence represent greater immediate threats to sex workers than acquisition of HIV and other STI. Sex workers also may "downgrade" their sense of personal risk from activities they otherwise acknowledge as potentially hazardous as a psychological coping mechanism (Varga, 2001).

Efforts to design and implement sexual health interventions for sex workers thus need to holistically explore sex workers' experience in each specific context, including understanding what one author has called the "local cultural logic" of risk (Hanson, Lopez-Iftikhar & Alegria, 2002, p. 292). Only when sex workers can address their communities' priority issues, as in the Sonagachi movement, will they be able to consider less imminent threats such as HIV. Against this backdrop, the study described below aimed to engage with sex workers' own worldview and to position the design of interventions within their understandings of risks in their lives.

The context of this study is the brothel district of Svay Pak, Cambodia, in which over 300 Vietnamese migrant women live and sell sex. Brothel-based sex work was identified early in Cambodia's epidemic as one of the primary routes of transmission (Pisani et al., 2003). In the mid-1990s, some populations of sex workers exhibited prevalence rates reaching 40% (Ryan et al., 1998) although national estimates suggested that approximately one-third were infected (NCHADS, 2000). In response, the government launched a 100% condom campaign targeting brothels modeled on the Thai policy. Recent figures show that although the national adult prevalence has dropped from close to 4% to 2.7%, levels of HIV have remained at 31.1% of brothel-based sex workers (UNAIDS, 2002b).

Svay Pak is one of the largest and best-known brothel districts, located on the outskirts of Cambodia's capital, Phnom Penh. Traditionally a fishing village and long-term Vietnamese community, Svay Pak is better known for its two main streets lined by over 20 brothels. Young women migrate from southern Vietnam to escape sustained rural poverty and earn money for their families; some seek an independent lifestyle or flee difficult personal circumstances (Busza, 2004). Upon arrival, each woman enters an agreement with a specific brothel. The managers pay an advance fee, ranging from U.S. $50 to $3000, to the sex worker, her relatives or community intermediaries. Through an established debt system, the sex worker pays back this sum through her work, servicing an average of 15 clients per week over a period of six to eighteen months (Baker et al., 2001).

The sex workers in Cambodia are in a doubly marginalised position as they are illegal immigrants working in a criminalized occupation. As such, they are vulnerable to abuse and exploitation. Police and local military authorities harass brothel managers and sex workers by extorting "protection money," demanding free sexual services, and conducting arrests. Brothel managers maintain strict control over sex workers' mobility, in part to avoid arrests but also to maximize productivity and reduce the chances that a sex worker will leave the brothel without paying her debt. Sex workers generally stay inside the brothel waiting for clients. They have few opportunities to socialize with others outside their own brothels as managers view competing establishments with suspicion. Competition between brothels and between individual women also puts pressure on sex workers to agree to clients' demands.

METHODS

Participants and Procedures

The research presented here forms part of an evaluation study of a community empowerment project conducted by Medecins Sans Frontieres/Belgium (MSF), "Building community identity among debt-bonded Vietnamese sex workers in Cambodia." Data collection and analysis were conducted under the auspices of the Population Council's Horizons program in local collaboration with Cambodian Researchers for Development (CRD). The project ran from April 2000 through March 2002.

MSF implemented a social intervention to expand its clinic-based services for sex workers. Although the clinic had offered primary health care, syndromic management, condom promotion, and counseling to the Svay Pak community since the mid-1990s, staff increasingly realized that sex workers faced barriers to safeguarding their health that could not be overcome through improved medical care or individual-level knowledge. To address structural factors shaping sex workers' vulnerability, MSF launched the "Lotus Club," a safe, social space located upstairs from the clinic where sex workers could relax and meet each other. The development, aims, and objectives of this intervention have been described in greater detail elsewhere (Busza & Schunter, 2001). Trained Vietnamese-speaking facilitators conducted regular participatory discussions for small groups in order to establish community identity, strengthen solidarity between sex workers, and stimulate critical analysis and collective action. These sessions based interactive activities around topics such as saving money, feeling homesick, developing supportive networks, and negotiating safer sexual behaviors with clients and boyfriends. Sex workers suggested many of the topics discussed and over the course of the intervention recommended, then selected, additional project activities such as foreign language classes.

Evaluation methods were integrated into the intervention. All participatory discussion activities with sex workers were documented and analyzed, including diagrams, charts, and group discussions, as well as the facilitators' observations and comments. In total, over 300 sex workers participated in organized participatory workshops over the two-year period, covering 25 different topics. Each workshop lasted approximately two hours and involved between 6 and 10 participants. These sessions proved extremely popular, particularly for offering the opportunity for women to meet peers from other brothels with whom they ordinarily had almost no contact, and for addressing serious topics in an informal, entertaining manner.

The use of participatory and interactive methods for both research and practice encourages participants to control both process and content of elicited information, emphasizing community "voices" over researchers' own knowledge (Pretty, Gujit, Thompson & Scoones, 1995, Shah, Kambou & Monahan, 1999). As an approach, participatory research also strengthens critical analysis and communication skills through its emphasis on interactive activities, which position community members as agents of social change rather than passive recipients of "best practice" (Ford & Koetsawang, 1999). The data presented in this paper draw on these methods and are analyzed specifically in regard to sex workers' own interpretations of risks in their lives and work, with subsequent discussion of the implications for future interventions for brothel-based sex workers.

RESULTS

Figure 1 offers a comprehensive overview of how sex workers in Svay Pak conceptualized the challenges of life and work in the community, drawn by a group of 6 participants six months after the project started. Other groups produced remarkably similar diagrams when conducting the same activity. Some of the most salient themes regarding perceptions of "risk," therefore, emerged early in the study.

The diagram demonstrates the holistic way in which sex workers in Svay Pak viewed occupational hazards. They identified a range of concerns rooted in both the causes and consequences of their participation in prostitution. Although sexual health risks, including pregnancy, unsafe abortion, STI and HIV, featured among the highlighted problems, they were embedded in a more comprehensive understanding of risk and not necessarily prioritized. This activity found that sex workers also feared uncooperative, drunk or violent clients, abusive police authori-

FIGURE 1

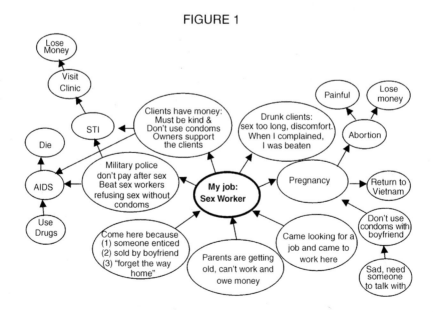

ties, and demanding brothel managers. They experienced economic pressures from family members in Vietnam. Loneliness, the need for personal relationships, and seeking independence from traditional rural life (sometimes referred to as "forgetting the way home") also contributed to negative outcomes.

These findings were further reflected in other activities, interviews, and discussions conducted with sex workers in Svay Pak over the two-year intervention, as presented below. When characterizing their motivations and concerns, sex workers voiced a clear hierarchy. Above all, they prioritized fulfilling obligations to their families by helping meet economic needs. Any threats to their ability to achieve this were viewed as primary risks in their lives. As a result, sex workers specifically tried to avoid disruption, persecution and violence, and aimed to maintain emotional and physical well-being.

Fulfilling Family Obligations

The majority of women in Svay Pak migrated from southern Vietnam to earn money and contribute to their families' livelihoods through short-term sex work. Sex workers repeatedly stressed the importance of maximizing their incomes in order to help alleviate their families' poverty. In some cases, they aspired to pay off their debt to the brothel as quickly as possible and return to Vietnam, while others remained for longer periods, hoping to regularly forward earnings home. In both cases, the number of clients and payments received remained a chief preoccupation and dominated thoughts and conversations.

While this concern for meeting the family's financial needs could contribute to a sex worker's anxiety, it also served as a source of pride in the important role she played in her household's survival, and in her ability to create opportunities for the future. This pride could somewhat mitigate perceived difficulties and risks inherent to sex work:

> *My family is poor, that is why I have to come here to work. I have to work. I have to help my brothers or sisters go to school. Sex work is hard work, there are drunk clients, intercourse is hard and long and makes me hurt. I'm scared of AIDS, sometimes the condoms break during intercourse. . . . [but] I want to earn money and go back to Vietnam to run a coffee shop to support my young brothers and sisters. (age 20, working 6 months)*

Prioritizing future ambitions led sex workers to make rational choices that could jeopardize their health. In order to make as much money as possible, sex workers accepted all available clients and often did not feel able to negotiate condom use lest they lose customers to competing peers. Sex workers also actively sought out foreign clients who paid higher fees set by the brothels, and had a reputation for tipping generously, although they also proved least likely to agree to use condoms:

> *When I'm going out with Japanese clients, USA clients, Chinese clients, I'm very happy because they tip me a lot of money and I can pay off my debt very soon. Sometimes they treat me very bad, [or] they don't use condoms. But I'm not afraid of disease, just think about paying my debt soon. (age 20, working 12 months)*

Few sex workers in Svay Pak proved naïve or poorly informed regarding the presence of HIV and STI in the community; several could name sex workers who had fallen ill and returned to die in Vietnam. Figure 1 also bears testament to the complex understanding sex workers exhibited in relation to a wide range of interlinked social, physical, and emotional problems. Sex workers were not ignorant of these risks, therefore, but rather adopted a coping strategy of minimizing or disregarding negative sexual health outcomes in order to preserve a focus on meeting their economic goals, as summarized by this participant:

> *I have to work and pay off my debt. If I am worried about my health then I cannot earn money–who will give me money? (age 18, working 7 months)*

At the most extreme, some sex workers developed a fatalistic attitude, disavowing hope for the future while elevating their need to fulfill family obligations to an overarching life purpose:

> *I'm a sex worker and I don't think anything at all. I just want to earn money for my family. If I get diseases and die it is not problem. (age 16, worked 7 months)*

Although the above statement is an exception rather than the norm, reflecting the deepest levels of depression found in Svay Pak, it demonstrates the way in which sex workers' primary aim–that of making money for their families in Vietnam–could eclipse most other concerns.

Those that did retain importance to sex workers generally represented threats to their ability to work and earn, and are addressed below.

Avoiding Persecution and Violence

Police harassment remained a persistent problem for both sex workers and brothel owners in Svay Pak. In addition to paying regular "protection money" to local authorities, the community was at the mercy of a range of police forces, including those from the nearby capital, and the particularly feared military police. The Phnom Penh police tended to conduct brothel raids and arrests, often to supplement their incomes through bribes paid to secure the release of sex workers or managers from custody. The military police, on the other hand, terrorized the community, often through drunken rampages involving violence, threats, and demands for sex without pay. Throughout the study, sex workers' fear of police emerged as paramount:

> *Sometimes they [police] come to ask us for money for their phone card or petrol. They do not pay us for sex, ask us to have oral sex, change positions during sex, drink without paying. Raids. We have to pay [bribes] to get back. . . . I'm very scared of them, whenever I see them coming to raid other brothels, I always run to the taxi driver's house to hide. (Age 17, working 8 months)*

> *Drunk police come with guns and if they refuse to use a condom, the sex worker must agree. The sex workers are afraid of being shot, and also afraid that the police will smash up the brothel. (Group activity on work conditions)*

In addition to the obvious physical risks of police abuse, raids and arrests added bribery costs to sex workers' debts, thereby increasing the time spent working in brothels and heightening the urgency to maximize client numbers, particularly the best-paying ones. Furthermore, the disruption caused by police activity reduced clientele, especially when police launched a series of crackdowns ostensibly to close the industry altogether. Usually, after a few days or weeks during which sex workers either operated secretly behind locked doors or were sent away to await better times, business in Svay Pak would return to normal. In the meantime, however, sex workers experienced severe loss of income while incurring additional costs:

> *At the moment, police are coming around Svay Pak and all of the brothels have to close, [there are] no clients. . . . Now that there are not so many clients, [we] can't earn money to spend for the New Year and no money to send back home. (Group activity on recent changes in the community)*

Persecution and violence by police left sex workers feeling extremely vulnerable, and further reduced their ability to control work conditions. These threats also exacerbated sex workers' anxieties over not securing sufficient income to meet family needs or repay debts, making them more likely to take other risks.

Maintaining Well-Being

The third theme that emerged in sex workers' descriptions of life and work in Svay Pak related to safeguarding their own physical, emotional, and mental well-being. Here sex workers stated worries around risks to sexual and reproductive health, fearing STI, including HIV/AIDS, and unwanted pregnancy, which invariably resulted in illegal and possibly unsafe abortions. Yet these risks were embedded within more general health concerns. Sex workers listed a range of occupational hazards:

> *We stay up late and don't eat healthy food and then lose money to buy medicine. We need to rest, not work overtime, eat health food and use medicine. (Group activity on general health)*

Many study participants emphasized the importance of looking after themselves, however, and preserving good health to prevent taking time off work and losing income through a reduction in clients or through the costs of medicines and other treatment.

> *Health is very important, if we have good health then we can work and earn money, and if we earn money then we can have a free life so we can go back to live with our families. (Group activity on work conditions)*

Sex workers often expressed a sense that Svay Pak was not a healthy environment; rather, it was unstable, often dangerous, and amoral. Although the women viewed their stay in the community as both temporary and necessary, they voiced the need to actively preserve their well-being to survive the precariousness around them:

Social life here is very complicated, disordered. Vietnamese and Khmer people mix together. A lot of people are infected with AIDS, here there are many gamblers, many people drink alcohol, there is fighting–and the police never solve the problems. Police arrest the sex workers. Life here has no value. (Group activity on life in Svay Pak)

[I] feel sometimes good and sometimes bad, because my friends go out with other people and my boyfriend had another girl. So when I feel sad, I like to go to the café shop and sit there alone. (Group activity on relationships within the community)

As the quote above intimates, one strategy adopted by some sex workers to mitigate the emotional pitfalls of their work was to cultivate personal romantic relationships. The nature of these relationships varied, with some sex workers developing romantic ties with their regular customers, while others forged relationships outside their work and appeared to manage to hide their occupation. Boyfriends represented a source of support, affection, and occasionally hope for the future.

I like to go out and like to have a boyfriend because I need love. (group activity on positives and negatives in Svay Pak)

Although most sex workers acknowledged that boyfriends could only serve an immediate emotional need, some aspired to a more permanent union, and possible a new life somewhere else, particularly if the boyfriend came from abroad. One Japanese client arranged a passport for his girlfriend so she could accompany him home on holidays. In rare cases, clients maintained long-term relationships or married sex workers:

I have an American boyfriend, we have known each other for over one year. In April last year he helped me to apply for a visa to go to the USA, now I got a visa for 5 years. He promises to come and see me next month and we [will] go to the USA together. (age 21, working 36 months)

Not all sex workers found romantic relationships a useful coping strategy, however, as it could prove distracting from a single minded focus on earning money or introduce complications:

I'm a sex worker and I don't love clients. Clients have money to buy sex. I don't have any sentiment with clients. (age 20, working 12 months)

There is evidence that due to the supportive and emotional role served by boyfriends, sex workers tended to waive their attempts to negotiate safer sex. As indicated through one of the pathways in the diagram presented earlier, feeling sad and lonely could lead to not using a condom with boyfriends, resulting in pregnancy. That STI or HIV does not appear to feature in this pathway springs from sex workers' downgrading of risks posed by boyfriends:

This month I had sex with my boyfriend without a condom one time. At first he used a condom, but during intercourse I asked him to take the condom off because he was drunk and intercourse was taking a long time. . . . I think my boyfriend is very young and he is a student, maybe he doesn't have any diseases, I don't know. (age 18, working 7 months)

In these cases, therefore, the perception that fostering personal and romantic relationships could alleviate sex workers' risks of anxiety and loneliness caused sex workers to deemphasize other risks, such as vulnerability to infection.

DISCUSSION

As seen, sex workers in Svay Pak positioned sexual and reproductive health concerns within a wider understanding of the risks faced through sex work. Their perceptions and interpretations, therefore, will affect response to public health interventions, such as HIV prevention messages advocating individual behavior change. Women in Svay Pak were familiar with risks such as HIV, STI, and unwanted pregnancy and knew how to prevent them. Yet given the complex tangle of occupational risks, they adopted strategies to meet immediate needs that did not always prioritize seeking to avoid STI and HIV.

Sex workers' main concern was ensuring financial gain and contributing to the livelihoods of their families. To achieve this and maximize their ability to work unimpeded, sex workers strove to mitigate disruption and harassment by police, and to maintain their emotional and physical well-being. Attitudes to sexual health risks were shaped by these driving motivations, and thus can only be understood when seen through sex workers' own world view. Within this, behaviors that are "risky" from a sexual health perspective such as accepting all clients, including those who refuse to wear condoms, or seeking romantic relationships that also involve unprotected sex, proved to be rational choices, and indeed, risk-reduction measures if a more holistic understanding of "risk" is used.

Although this renders traditional HIV prevention tactics more challenging, working within sex workers' own reality can offer more feasible and sustainable opportunities for change. For example, sex workers' mixed feelings regarding hopes for their futures could be harnessed for health promotion. Although some women appeared to adopt a fatalistic approach to their work, many sex workers viewed their participation in the sex industry as a short-term necessity that brought crucial assistance to their families and assured a brighter future for themselves. As they themselves acknowledged, remaining healthy was a prerequisite for achieving their economic goals and realizing dreams for the future. Interventions could thus take a wider view of health and work with the community to facilitate analysis of how to balance short term needs with longer-term aspirations, and what new safeguards might be feasible. Building critical life skills such as enhancing sex workers' capacity to save money or plan realistic goals might also help them maximize their incomes through new strategies, and reevaluate the opportunity costs of shorter-term approaches.

Similarly, addressing emotional relationships too often gets left out of HIV prevention messages. Although sex workers are often encouraged to negotiate safer practices with clients, their intimate interactions with boyfriends or regular clients usually do not get the same attention. In Svay Pak, although some women aspired to leaving sex work for a new life with an intimate partner, more commonly boyfriends represented a temporary comfort and outlet for emotional needs. Sex workers often complained that it was difficult to mix or make friends outside the brothel, and that they suffered from boredom. Offering sex workers other means of psycho-social support and opportunities for rest, leisure activity, and social interaction with one another could contribute to a reduction in dependence on boyfriends. This could be coupled with improving negotiation and communication skills, focusing on personal rather than commercial interactions, and could perhaps include participation of boyfriends in activities as well.

Mitigating the risks at the forefront of sex workers' analytical framework, therefore, could shift their importance within the risk environment, potentially creating space for sex workers to address the currently less pressing concerns of sexual health and HIV prevention. Sustained participatory engagement with a given community on a wide range of issues offers an entry point into sex workers' worldview, enabling the development of intervention strategies tackling a holistic experience of risk, rather than retaining a narrow epidemiological focus unlikely to effect sustainable behavior change.

Ultimately, however, prevention efforts need to engage with the much more difficult structural parameters of risk within commercial sex in Cambodia including criminalization of the industry, lack of accountability within police forces, and the often exploitative control wielded by brothel managers. The legal status of sex work is perhaps the most critical, as it blurs the line between police harassment and law enforcement. Furthermore, sex workers had no access to legal redress for exploitation or human rights abuses experienced at the hands of authorities, brothel management, or clients. As both illegal immigrants from Vietnam and engaged in an illegal form of labor, they cannot shape work on their own terms. Until these fundamental limitations on sex workers' control over their lives are removed, it is difficult to imagine a reshaping of their interpretations and responses to risks that currently can exacerbate rather than reduce vulnerability to HIV.

Due to their occupational exposure to multiple sexual partners and low condom use, sex workers have often been identified as a primary "risk group" for the transmission of HIV in many settings. Although programmatic focus has shifted from individual behavior change interventions to addressing structural determinants of sex workers' vulnerability, most public health efforts continue to target behavioral "risks" as defined by epidemiological approaches to HIV/AIDS prevention. Sex workers themselves, however, are likely to view their experiences more holistically, perceiving a range of risks confronting them through their work. Although they may acknowledge the same sexual and reproductive health risks as public health professionals, they may not prioritize them in the same way.

This qualitative study among Vietnamese sex workers in Svay Pak, Cambodia, found a clear hierarchy of concerns within the community. Sex workers took pride in their ability to contribute to their families' incomes and viewed their role as earners as of foremost importance. Threats to the potential to fulfill these obligations proved among sex workers' most serious preoccupations and led them to adopt various strategies including maximizing numbers of clients and choosing clients who paid well but often refused to use condoms. Fear of police harassment ranked second in sex workers' fears, due to its violence, destabilization, and disruption to normal work conditions. Finally, and intimately linked to the first two characterizations of risk, sex workers described how life in Svay Pak could be detrimental to their well-being, by inducing anxiety, loneliness, and poor physical and psycho-social health.

This conceptual framework voiced by the sex worker community highlights how behavioral risk factors related to HIV transmission and acquisition can be embedded in a more complex understanding of risk. Indeed, the means through which sex workers attempted to reduce these threats could actually exacerbate their vulnerability, despite good awareness of the epidemic, other sexual health problems, and how to prevent them. In order to specifically address sexual behavioral risks, therefore, interventions need to comprehensively understand not just the conditions of the local sex industry, but also how sex worker communities perceive, interpret and react to them. Subsequent design and implementation of risk-reduction activities could thus be based on sex workers' own experiences, aspirations, and existing coping strategies, using them as a realistic entry point for efforts to change both individual behaviors and community-level structures.

REFERENCES

Asthana, S. & Oostvogels, R. (1996). Community participation in HIV prevention: Problems and prospects for community-based strategies among female sex workers in Mafra. *Social Science and Medicine, 43*, 133-148.

Baker, S., Busza, J., Tienchantuk, P., Ly, S. D., Un, S., Hom, E. X. & Schunter, B. T. (2001). Promotion of community identification and participation in community activities in a population of debt-bonded sex workers in Svay Pak. 6th *International Congress on AIDS in Asia and the Pacific*, 5-10 October, Melbourne, Australia.

Busza, J. & Schunter, B. T. (2001). From competition to community: participatory learning and action among young, debt-bonded Vietnamese sex workers in Cambodia. *Reproductive Health Matters, 9*, 72-81.

Busza, J. (2004). Sex work and migration: the dangers of oversimplification. *Health and Human Rights, 7*, 231-250.

Campbell, C. (2000). Selling sex in the time of AIDS: the psycho-social context of condom use by sex workers on a Southern African mine. *Social Science and Medicine, 50*, 479-494.

Campbell, C. (2003). *Letting them Die: Why HIV/AIDS Prevention Programmes Fail.* Oxford: International African Institute in association with James Curry.

Campbell, C. & Mzaidume, Z. (2001). Grassroots participation, peer education, and HIV prevention by sex workers in South Africa. *American Journal of Public Health, 91*, 1978-1986.

Day, S. & Ward, H. (1997). Sex workers and the control of sexually transmitted disease. *Genitourinary Medicine*, *73*, 161-168.

Fontanet, A. L., Saba, J., Chandelying, V., Sakondhavat, C., Bhiraleus, P., Rugpao, S. et al. (1998). Protection against sexually transmitted diseases by granting sex workers in Thailand the choice of using the male or female condom: results from a randomized control trial. *AIDS*, *12*, 1851-1859.

Ford, N. J. & Koetsewang, S. (1999). Narrative explorations and self-esteem: research, intervention and policy of HIV prevention in the sex industry in Thailand. *International Journal of Population Geography*, *5*, 213-233.

Ford, K., Wirawan, D. N., Reed, B. D., Muliawan, P. & Wolfe, R. (2002). The Bali STD/AIDS study: Evaluation of an intervention for sex workers. *Sexually Transmitted Diseases*, *29*, 50-58.

Hanenberg, R., Rojanapithayakorn, W., Kunasol, P. & Sokal, D. (1994). Impact of Thailand's HIV-control programme as indicated by the decline of sexually transmitted diseases. *Lancet*, *344*, 243-245.

Hanson, H., Lopez-Iftikhar, M. M. & Alegria, M. (2002). The economy of risk and respect: accounts by Puerto Rican sex workers of HIV risk taking. *The Journal of Sex Research*, *39*, 292-301.

Jana, S., Bandyopadhyay, Mukherjee, S., Dutta, N., Basu, I. & Saha, A. (1998). STD/HIV intervention with sex workers. *AIDS*, *12*, S101-S108.

Joesoef, M., Kio, D., Linnan, M., Kamboji, A., Barakbah, Y. & Idajadi, A. (2000). Determinants of condom use in female sex workers in Surabaya, Indonesia. *International Journal of STDs and AIDS*, *11*, 262-265.

Lau, J. T. F., Tsui, H. Y., Siah, P. C. & Zhang, K. L. (2002). A study on female sex workers in southern China (Shenzhen): HIV-related knowledge, condom use and STD history. *AIDS Care*, *14*, 219-233.

Loff, B., Overs, C. & Longo, P. (2003). Can health programmes lead to mistreatment of sex workers? *Lancet*, *361*, 1982-3.

NCHADS (2000). *Executive Summary of the Results of HIV Sentinel Surveillance 1999 in Cambodia*. Phnom Penh: National Centre for HIV/AIDS, Dermatology and STDs.

NSWP (1997). *Making Sex Work Safe*. London: Network of Sex Work Projects.

Parker, R. G., Easton, D. & Klein, C. H. (2000). Structural barriers and facilitators in HIV prevention: a review of international research. *AIDS*, *14*, S22-S32.

Pauw, I. & Brener, L. (2003). "You are just whores–you can't be raped": barriers to safer sex practices among women street sex workers in Cape Town. *Culture, Health & Sexuality*, *5*, 465-481.

Pisani, E., Garnett, G. P., Brown, T., Stover, J., Grassly, N. C., Hankins, C. et al. (2003). Back to basics in HIV prevention: focus on exposure. *BMJ*, *326*, 1384-7.

Plummer, F. A., Nagelkerke, N. J., Moses, S., Ndinya-Achola, J. O., Bwayo, J. & Ngugi, E. (1991). The importance of core groups in the epidemiology and control of HIV-1 infection. *AIDS*, *5 Suppl 1*, S169-76.

Pretty, J. N., Gujit, I., Thompson, J. & Scoones, I. (1995). *Participatory Learning and Action: A Trainer's Guide*. London: IIED.

Ray, S., van de Wijgert, J., Mason, P., Ndowa, F. & Maposhere, C. (2001). Constraints faced by sex workers in use of female and male condoms for safer sex in urban Zimbabwe. *Journal of Urban Health, 78*, 581-592.

Ryan, C. A., Ouk, V. V., Gorbach, P. M., Leng, H. B., Berlioz-Arthaud, A., Whittington, W. & Holmes, K. K. (1998). Explosive spread of HIV-1 and sexually transmitted diseases in Cambodia. *The Lancet, 351*, 1175.

Shah, M. K., Kambou, S. D. & Monahan, B. (1999). *Embracing Participation in Development.* Atlanta: CARE.

Tawil, O., O'Reilly, K., Coulibaly, I.-M., Tiemele, A., Himmich, H., Boushaba, A., Pradeep, K. & Carael, M. (1999). HIV prevention among vulnerable populations: outreach in the developing world. *AIDS, 13*, S239-S247.

UNAIDS (1996). *The Status and Trends of the Global HIV/AIDS Pandemic.* Vancouver: Official Satellite Symposium, UNAIDS and AIDSCAP/FHI.

UNAIDS (2002a). *Report on the Global HIV/AIDS Epidemic 2002.* Geneva: Joint United National Programme on HIV/AIDS (UNAIDS).

UNAIDS (2002b). *Cambodia Epidemiological Fact Sheet on HIV/AIDS and Sexually Transmitted Infections.* Geneva: Joint UN Programme on HIV/AIDS (UNAIDS).

Varga, (2001). Coping with HIV/AIDS in Durban's commercial sex industry. *AIDS Care, 13*, 351-665.

Wojcicki, J. M. & Malala, J. (2001). Condom use, power and HIV/AIDS risk: sex workers bargain for survival in Hillbrow/Joubert Park/Berea, Johannesburg. *Social Science and Medicine, 53*, 99-121.

Wolffers, I. & van Beelen, N. (2003). Public health and the human rights of sex workers. *Lancet, 361*, 1981.

Wong, M. L., Lubek, I., Dy, B. C., Pen, S., Kros, S. & Chhit, M. (2003). Social and behavioral factors associated with condom use among direct sex workers in Siem Reap, Cambodia. *Sexually Transmitted Infections, 79*, 163-165.

Female Sex Trade Workers, Condoms, and the Public-Private Divide

Lois A. Jackson, PhD
Barbara Sowinski, BPR
Carolyn Bennett
Devota Ryan, MSW

SUMMARY. This qualitative study explored the ways in which social relations within the public (work) as opposed to the private (home) contexts shape variable condom use among female sex trade workers. Semi-structured interviews were conducted with 68 female sex workers

Lois A. Jackson and Barbara Sowinski are affiliated with Dalhousie University, Nova Scotia.

Carolyn Bennett is affiliated with the Stepping Stone Association, Nova Scotia.

Devota Ryan is affiliated with the Region 7 Hospital Corporation, New Brunswick.

Address correspondence to: Lois A. Jackson, School of Health and Human Performance, Dalhousie University, 6230 South Street, Halifax, Nova Scotia, Canada B3H 3J5 (E-mail: Lois.jackson@dal.ca).

The authors would like to thank the research assistants on this study, Colleen Whyte, Amy Kwok, Camille Dumond and Chrystie Myketiak, for their assistance with the data management aspects of the study. Thanks also to Chrystie Myketiak for her careful proofreading. The authors also want to extend their sincere thanks and appreciation to all of the women who gave of their time and who volunteered for this study by telling their "story." The authors would also like to thank the Social Sciences and Humanities Research Council (SSHRCC) for the generous financial support that allowed them to conduct this research (Project # 410-98-0435). Lois A. Jackson is the recipient of an Investigator's Award through the Canadian Institutes of Health Research (CIHR), and would like to thank this funding agency for their support.

[Haworth co-indexing entry note]: "Female Sex Trade Workers, Condoms, and the Public-Private Divide." Jackson, Lois A. et al. Co-published simultaneously in *Journal of Psychology & Human Sexuality* (The Haworth Press, Inc.) Vol. 17, No. 1/2, 2005, pp. 83-105; and: *Contemporary Research on Sex Work* (ed: Jeffrey T. Parsons) The Haworth Press, Inc., 2005, pp. 83-105. Single or multiple copies of this article are available for a fee from The Haworth Document Delivery Service [1-800-HAWORTH, 9:00 a.m. - 5:00 p.m. (EST). E-mail address: docdelivery@haworthpress.com].

working in various settings in an urban center in Eastern Canada. The findings suggest that work-related social relations, and the meanings associated with condoms at work, create a strong confidence in condom use. Within the private setting, such confidence was also evident but most women reported either not using condoms or only using "sometimes." Nevertheless, many women do engage in risk management within the private setting, and take active steps to decrease their risks of Human Immunodeficiency Syndrome (HIV)/Sexually Transmitted Infections (STIs). *[Article copies available for a fee from The Haworth Document Delivery Service: 1-800-HAWORTH. E-mail address: <docdelivery@haworthpress.com> Website: <http://www.HaworthPress.com> © 2005 by The Haworth Press, Inc. All rights reserved.]*

KEYWORDS. Female sex trade workers, public-private divide, social relations, HIV/STIs, condom use

During the early years of the HIV pandemic, female sex trade workers were depicted as a source of the spread of HIV–as "vectors of transmission" to the heterosexual population (Alexander, 1997). In more recent years, public health concerns have focused on the risks female sex trade workers face while providing services to clients. Efforts have centered on the prevention of HIV within the trade, and as part of this prevention strategy numerous studies have examined the prevalence of condom use among sex trade workers as well as determinants of use. Within numerous North American and Australian cities, and parts of Europe, researchers have found high rates of condom use between female sex trade workers and their clients, especially when having anal or vaginal intercourse, with less consistent use for oral sex (Donegan, 1996; Green, Goldberg, Christie, Frischer, Thomson, Carr & Taylor, 1993; Jackson, Highcrest & Coates, 1992; Vanwesenbeech, van Zessen, DeGraaf & Straver, 1994; Venema & Visser, 1990).

Vanwesenbeeck et al.'s (1994) study of 119 female sex trade workers in the Netherlands, for example, revealed that 93 or 78% of the women surveyed used condoms consistently in vaginal or anal sex with clients. These researchers refer to the women as consistent protectors, and argue that, "The interaction between a prostitute and a client which results in unprotected sex can be considered a deviation from the standard interaction scenario in prostitution encounters" (1994, p.315). In a sample of female street workers in Glasgow, Green et al. (1993) report a similar pattern stating that the "typical" street worker has good knowledge of HIV/AIDS, and for vaginal intercourse almost always uses condoms with clients.

Condom use with clients is not new to the HIV era. Research with sex trade workers prior to the discovery of HIV reported use of condoms between female sex trade workers and their clients. McLeod (1982) noted that female prostitutes in England often insisted on the male client using a "rubber contraceptive," and that many women took great care not to contract venereal diseases out of "self interest and a general concern for other people's welfare" (p.55). Since the development of HIV, researchers have attempted to understand the specific determinants of condom use, including the contexts that shape nonuse, and the sub-populations within the sex trade industry who may be most vulnerable to the nonuse of condoms (Campbell, 2000; Erickson, Butters, McGillicuddy & Hallgren, 2000; Gavey, McPhillips, Doherty, 2001; Kinnell, 1991; Pyett & Warr, 1997; Sterk, 1999; Surratt, Wechsberg, Cottler & Leukefeld, 1998; Wojciki & Malala, 2001). Nevertheless, the spotlight has remained on female sex trade workers' working or commercial lives with relatively little attention given to the determinants of condom use with their non-paying partners. This is in spite of the fact that a number of researchers have suggested that there is less consistent condom use within female sex trade workers' private lives, and that non-paying partners are frequently at high risk of HIV through the use of injection drug paraphernalia (Dorfman, Derish & Cohen, 1992; Jackson et al., 1992; Jackson & Hood, 2001; McKeganey, Barnard & Bloor, 1990; McKeganey & Barnard, 1992; Pyett & Warr, 1997; Surratt et al., 1998; Sterk, 1999; Venema & Visser, 1990; Weiner, 1996). Pyett and Warr (1997) found high levels of condom use between female sex workers and clients in Australia, but only about one-third of respondents indicated using condoms with their private or non-commercial partners. Alexander (1997, p.89) concurs that female sex trade workers are at risk of HIV infection, and the risk is typically not "prostitution per se," but rather, private sexual relations. Scambler, Peswani, Renton and Scambler (1990) further note that a paradoxical situation seems to exist in that female sex trade workers may become infected with HIV from contact with their boyfriend or lover, but clients may remain free from infection because of sex trade workers' use of condoms at work.

A greater understanding of condom use/nonuse within female sex trade workers' private lives is needed to assist in the development of programs aimed at targeting this potentially high risk area of women's lives. Our research seeks to provide insight into the ways in which context or setting (i.e., the public and private spheres), shapes condom use practices among these women. The intent of the research is to highlight the ways in which social relations, and different contexts of relationships between female sex trade workers and others, shape condom use and the meanings attached to condoms. The study is not aimed at quantifying the extent to which condoms are or are not used. Rather, using the principles of grounded theory and based on thematic analysis of sex trade workers' stories of condom use, the main goal is to inform our knowledge of how contextual influences can shape health-related practices and the meanings associated with those practices.

This paper is based on data collected from women who work in many different venues, and therefore, we have been able to examine condom use for a broad spectrum of women who work in the sex trade rather than only women who work on the streets. With some notable exceptions (Jesson, Luck & Taylor, 1994; Lian, Chan & Wee, 2000; Maticka-Tyndale & Lewis, 1999), much of the information about female sex trade workers has historically been limited to street working women because of the visibility of this group of women, and the relatively easier access to these women (Barnard, 1993; Dalla, 2000; Youth Services Bureau, 1991).

METHODS

Participants and Procedure

Sixty-nine female sex trade workers living at the time in Halifax, Nova Scotia, were interviewed for this study. (Halifax is located in the Eastern part of the country, and is a port city with a population of just over 300,000). One of the 69 interviews was considered lost because the woman could not attend to the questions asked. Therefore, 68 interviews were analyzed for this paper. All of the sex trade workers were interviewed at the office of a street outreach program for sex trade workers, and in a space that ensured confidentiality. The women were recruited through posters displayed at the street outreach program, advertisements in a local newspaper, and via word of mouth or a "snowball technique" in which women who had been interviewed told other women about the study. The women signed a consent form at the time of the interview, and were provided a small honorarium to help defray costs associated with being interviewed including lost income from not working, transportation and/or babysitting costs. The research protocol was reviewed and approved by the Ethics Committee at the University where the principal investigator of the study is a faculty member.

All interviews were conducted by the female principal investigator, a sociologist with years of interview experience. Near the end of each interview, the interview guide was scanned to ensure the woman had discussed all areas. If it was felt that an area required further elaboration, or had not been discussed by the respondent, further questions were asked.

Each interview lasted approximately 1 hour and 30 minutes. The guide provided an outline of the areas for discussion but allowed the women flexibility to discuss their "story" in a manner that made most sense to them. The 68 women ranged in age from 19 to 48 years with a mean age of 31. (See Table 1 for a summary of the socio-demographics of the women). All had been involved in the sex trade at some point in the year prior to the interview. Of the 68 women, 26 reported that they had worked on the streets and as an escort over the course of their career as a prostitute, 18 exclusively as a street prostitute, and 8 as an escort only (i.e., working for an escort service). The remaining 16 women reported working in various other settings and in various combinations of settings such as in bars, on the street, and out of their home.

With the exception of one interview, all interviews were audiotaped. This one interview was with a woman who was deaf and the interview was conducted by writing the questions, and the woman wrote her responses that were then analyzed as per the other interviews. The research assistants transcribed the audiotaped interviews verbatim.

Interview Questions

A semi-structured interview guide based on the research literature was initially developed by the research team and then reviewed by two sex trade workers who made suggestions for additional questions or probes, as well as the wording and placement of questions. The interviews began with general questions about the women's lives (e.g., age, where born, any children, etc.) and then asked about their working lives (e.g., when and why started, primary venue of work, relations with clients and others in the sex trade, etc.). The final section of the interview focused on the women's private relationships (e.g., how long together, nature of relationship, how it is the same or different from relationship with clients, etc.), and relationships with family and friends, as well as other community members. A specific area of interest was the use/non-use of condoms within the women's working and private lives and the

TABLE 1. Respondents' Socio-Demographics (N = 68)

Age at time of interview
Mean Age – 31 years (N = 67)

Age	Number	%
<20	1	2
20-29	27	40
30-39	33	49
40-48	6	9

Age when began working in the sex trade
(N = 67)

Age	Number	%
<20	38	57
=/>20	29	43

Highest level of education attained
N = 57

Education Level	Number	%
<Grade 12	29	50
<Grade 12 with non-specific upgrade	6	11
= Grade 12 or equivalent	8	14
>Post-secondary training/trade	13	23
Currently in high school	1	2

Location(s) in which work/have worked

Location	Number	%*
Escort Agency	8	12
Streets	18	27
Escort/Streets	26	38
Other Combinations/Locations[1]	16	24

* Numbers do not add up to 100% because of rounding error

[1]Other locations included bars, massage parlours, own home, etc. Other combinations refer to various locations other than exclusively escort agencies/streets.

women's understanding of why condoms are used/not used. It is this aspect of the interview that is the focus of this paper.

Data Analysis

All transcribed interviews were coded using a coding scheme developed by one of the research assistants and the principal investigator of the study, and according to the principles of grounded theory (Strauss, 1987). The coded interviews were placed in the NUDIST software program, which is a program for the management of qualitative data. A "report" of the women's narratives concerning condom use/non-condom use was prepared. The report was then analyzed for sub-themes according to the nature of the relationship (i.e., clients versus other sexual relationships), and relationships between sub-themes posited. The sub-themes and relationships between them were compared and contrasted for similarities and differences using the constant comparative process described by Strauss (1987) for the analysis of qualitative data. This process continued until saturation of concepts or no new concepts emerged from the data. The findings are reported using terms such as "a few," "some" and "many." This is because of the potential for numbers to be misinterpreted as representative of the entire population of sex trade workers.

RESULTS

The Work Context: Condoms a Must–Most of the Time

An analysis of the women's discussions concerning the use of condoms at work indicates not only that most of the women typically use condoms with clients, particularly when having vaginal or anal intercourse, but also that many are very confident of their ability to maintain condom use. Even if the client is a regular client, and there is a more familiar relationship than with other clients, the women reported that condoms remain high on their list of priorities. A 39-year-old woman who has worked on both the streets and indoors as an escort emphasized the importance of condoms with all clients irrespective of the degree of familiarity that might change other aspects of the commercial relationship.

> *I always use a condom. I never give that [a]way with them because*
> *you do it once and then they expect it all the time so condoms are*
> *very much a must in my eyes. I fluctuate in price if they are a regu-*
> *lar and they might say to me "well how about a 30 today, can you*
> *slide me in or whatever," that's fine, I'll do that. I tell them you,*
> *you know, don't get carried away, don't make this a habit. . . .*

The confidence the women expressed in their ability to use condoms even extended to times when it was dangerous to insist on condom use. One 28 year old woman who reported working on the streets and as an escort recounted a time when she was threatened by a client, and therefore serviced him free of charge yet still insisted on condom use. Another woman who did not provide her age but indicated that she has worked on the streets, in escort services and in massage parlours, stated that she sometimes takes advantage of situations when the client does not want to use a condom to surreptitiously put on a condom, and after she has completed the service she educates the client about the importance of condoms.

> *I never go out with anybody without a condom. You get johns who*
> *want to go without condoms and I'll say yes but when they come in,*
> *I'll put the condom in my mouth while I'm talking to them and*
> *move the condom around while I'm getting into position so that*
> *when I do go down on them, the condom [is] going down. I don't*
> *let them touch afterwards and I do my thing, they come and then I*
> *let them know they had a condom on cause you get them to think . . .*
> *and I tell them it's just mind over matter. . . .*

Although most of the women insisted that condoms were used on a regular basis irrespective of client demands, there were a few drug using women, and one woman who reported that she had mental health problems, who indicated that they were not consistent users of condoms. Of the 68 women we interviewed, 29 reported drug use, and of these, 9 indicated that they do not always use condoms. The reasons for not using condoms included being "off" [on drugs], and/or providing oral sex only, and/or in need of extra money, and/or servicing someone they believed was clean (e.g., an older man). A 31-year-old woman who reported that she was a drug user explained her non-condom use as follows:

I even was off a couple of times so bad, needed my fix so bad, did-n't have any condom . . . that I did it [serviced a client] unpro-tected—and that's fucking scary shit, you know?

A 35-year-old woman who was trying to get into a recovery program in-dicated that she only provides oral sex, and only uses condoms some-times.

If they're young guys I usually do [use condoms]. If they're older men, they're married, no I don't see a specific reason to. You know, I don't swallow or anything like that, so I don't see a spe-cific reason.

A 28-year-old woman who works on the streets, and indicated that she is a casual drug user, was very candid about her non-condom use when providing oral sex but indicated that she typically uses condoms when having sexual intercourse—although not in all cases.

. . . if I have sexual intercourse, I will use condoms . . . there is one john that won't use them and I haven't seen him in a while but he won't use them . . . he doesn't like it . . . he's an older man, he's up in his 50s . . . he doesn't like to use them . . . and he hasn't given me anything yet, but I do take an awful chance.

A couple of the women who reported that they previously used drugs in-dicated that in the past they did not always use condoms when they were "off" on drugs.

The confidence that the majority of the women expressed vis-à-vis the use of condoms with clients appears to be part of, and to be influ-enced by, a general culture of condom use within the sex trade industry within this community. The women's discussions of their relations with others in the sex trade industry including other sex trade workers, "pimps" (or an individual who takes all or much of the woman's earn-ings and insists that she work to provide economic support), owners of escort agencies, as well as clients, point to a general acceptance of, and support for, the use of condoms. In fact, a few of the women spoke of not knowing how to use condoms until they entered the sex trade and were taught about use as part of their training.

And I was young and naïve, earlier in my years, not using con-doms. I guess I wasn't schooled enough on that, my Mom never

*told me. The only . . . the only way I knew about condoms is when I
started working and girls used to tell me, "You have to [use con-
doms]." * [28 year old–street/escort]

A 40 year old woman working on the streets spoke of how her boyfriend
taught her how to slip a condom on a client without the client knowing.

*So I left my boyfriend from Canada and I started going out with a
guy from Los Angeles so I started going out with him and he taught
me more . . . a bit more about the business. He taught me how to
put a safe on a guy without him knowing that it was on there right?*

Support for the use of condoms was also evident in terms of comments about many of the escort services as the following exchange with
a 31-year-old woman reveals.

*Respondent: . . . One time. A buddy tried to pull the condom off
right?*

Interviewer: So what happened?

*Respondent: Well he did pull the condom off and came inside. But
I went to the doctor and got checked right away and the whole nine
yards and it was fine. But he was never allowed to call that service
again. They're really good with their girls. They are extremely
good with their girls.*

Many of the women reported that "most clients" are accepting of
condom use, and one woman reported that she even had clients that
would take her to purchase a condom if she did not have one. Yet another women indicated that "Johns," at times, supplied her with
condoms.

*Well, I'd go to the corner store and buy individual ones and I just
didn't always use them cause I didn't have them and stuff. One of
my Johns would supply them and say "use them." Right "use them
or you're going to end up regretting it."* [28 year old–street].

Some of the women who have worked for an extended period of time
reported that even prior to HIV condoms were used although they may
not have been used as consistently for vaginal and/or anal intercourse as

they are today. According to these women, prior to the HIV epidemic, condoms were more of an "option," and used with male clients who the women suspected might have a sexually transmitted infection (STI).

> *Respondent: Condoms were optional . . . in the birdybath you found something that wasn't good.*

> *Interviewer: In the birdybath?*

> *Respondent: Yes, or, what you have to do is you have to take the client in the bathroom, didn't matter where–hotel, their place, wherever, you take them in the bathroom and you kinda lather up his balls type thing, right? And in the process of doing that you're stimulating him a little, right, and then you go from the base of the balls and pull his skin toward the head right, and look at the fluid that come out the end. If it was clear fluid you were pretty much your own doctor, if it was clear fluid, you were good to go, if it was cloudy or anything then you would say well you know I have to use one of these things, blah, blah, blah, you know, cause you wouldn't want to get yourself infected. . . . [35 year old–escort]*

The women referred to condoms with clients as necessary because of the clear health benefits related to condom use. In the work context, condoms were associated with one's health and staying free of STIs especially HIV, as well as not becoming pregnant.

> *When you're working, health wise, just always use a condom always, you know. It doesn't matter how much money they're going to offer you to, you know to not use the condom, always use one and with the safety. . . . [29 year old–street/escort]*

> *Oh I tell them they had to [wear a condom], but most men do these days, most men do. And most . . . a lot of the men that want to have a condom with blow jobs too and . . . but I always . . . for intercourse I always . . . and because I'm fertile so I never . . . cause oh god, if I ever got pregnant and that'd be horrible. . . . [36 year old–street/escort/massage]*

In some instances, health and safety were understood not only in terms of the woman's personal health but also in terms of the health of her family. Indeed, use of condoms was associated with the woman's ability to continue to care for her family and to maintain her role as the breadwinner. For some women, therefore, condoms took on an importance beyond the immediate client-prostitute relationship and were connected to the broader context of their lives.

> *. . . some of them [clients] try to slip if off [condom] and some try to come up with all these lines, "I'm clean and I promise, I'm married" and all that kind of stuff. I just don't want to hear it. I really don't care. I got a 3-month-old child to care for at night, and you know, and that's that.* [31 year old–street/escort]

A few of the women suggested that condoms were associated with the "professional prostitute" as opposed to the unprofessional prostitute who they defined as the heavy drug-using prostitutes who would do anything for money. The "addicts" were frequently spoken about as failing to use condoms as well as providing services below market-price, thus contributing to a general unprofessional way of behaving. One woman spoke of her own past practice of providing oral sex without a condom in order to support her drug habit.

> *Interviewer: What would you charge when you're on the street?*

> *Respondent: Depended on how bad I wanted the money. I used to . . . to say $30 for a blowjob and $60 for . . . it was, a condom was not an option for intercourse. . . . If they were humming and hawing I would say it's $20 with a condom and $30 without for a blowjob. . . .* [35 year old–street/escort]

The Private (Home) Context

A number of researchers have found most female sex trade workers report consistent condom use at work but not at "home" with private partners. Our study found a similar pattern as most women reported consistent condom use at work, particularly when having intercourse with a client, but less consistent condom use in the context of sexual relations with a partner or lover. The use of condoms within the work context with clients, and the nonuse of condoms within the context of private relations, and the seemingly contradictory nature of this dichotomy were evident in the words of one woman who discussed the nature of condom use with "one night stands."

Now that I think back about it, it was kinda crazy to be doing I mean some guy in a van who probably fooled around with a lot of people right but ... ? Yeah, so ... but it was kinda crazy, you know what I mean, cause you go out and meet somebody you know and you only just meet them and you didn't use a condom with them but you use them with a client. [43 year old–street/bars/massage]

In a few instances, condoms were used in the private sphere with a lover or boyfriend. One woman indicated that she always uses condoms even when with private partners as you "never know" who your partner was with years ago. The same confidence that was evident when she spoke about condom use at work existed when she spoke about relations with her partner.

Interviewer: Do you use condoms with your private partner?

Respondent: Oh yes.

Interviewer: So that doesn't make a difference, whether it's your private partner or a client ... you always use condoms?

Respondent: I think everybody should cause you never know these days if your partner [has] you know, or if he's been [with some-one] years before you met him or I met him. I always use a con-dom. . . . [44 years–street/escorts]

Some women spoke of "manipulating" their partner in order to ensure condom use, and the strategy of not "giving sex" to their partner unless condoms were used mirrored the practice of not servicing clients without the use of condoms.

Respondent: Well if he choose to object he just don't get no ass, so that's up to him, you know what I mean? Half the time they won't object.

Interviewer: So he's never given you a hard time about using condoms?

Respondent: No, not at all, not at all. [27 year old–street]

A few of the women spoke of resistance to the use of condoms on the part of a boyfriend or spouse. The women indicated that their partner would be offended at the idea of being "treated like a trick" since condom use is associated with clients, and condoms would be opposed in very clear terms. Speaking about her relationship with "pimps" one woman commented:

> . . . *the pimps, if you asked them to use a condom, you could get beat for that. They'd accuse you of thinking of them as tricks, so there was no condoms with them.* . . . [29 year old–street/escort].

The most common response when asked about condom use with private partners, however, was neither a "never use" nor "always use" response. Rather, the response was typically–sometimes. Many of the women spoke of the varied ways in which condoms entered into their sexual relations with private partners depending upon the nature and power dynamics of the particular relationship, as well as the woman's reading or understanding of the relationship. Relationships were defined differently depending upon several factors including how long the woman was with her partner or knew her partner, and an assessment of the partner's trustworthiness particularly in terms of a commitment to the relationship.

A common practice reported by many of the women was one of utilizing condoms during the early part of the relationship, allowing time for blood tests to determine if they and/or their partner was/were disease free. A 28-year-old woman who works on both the streets and as an escort spoke of how she used condoms "early" in her relationship with her boyfriend until she and her boyfriend had proof that they were disease-free at which time they stopped using condoms.

> . . . *when I first started seeing him we used condoms for about a year until we both got checked and re-checked and checked again. And when we stopped using condoms, a month later they told me I was pregnant, something that was never supposed to happen.*

Another woman who worked only as an escort commented,

> *Well . . . we both went and we got checked before, we both had all our tests done . . . before the condom came off. Now this must sound funny, but I'm monogamous. Yeah and so is he. As far as I know.* [27 year old–escort]

In at least one instance, the woman's trust in her partner was based on having known him for a long period of time prior to becoming intimately involved, and knowing his past partner because they were part of the same community. One woman discussed her Hepatitis C status with her partner, and they mutually agreed to have sexual relations without a condom.

> *I've known him [boyfriend] for a lot of years anyways so the first time that we had sex it was like "are you clean . . . you've got nothing?" I said "no, you know I got Hep C" and he knew that anyways so . . . but you know it can't be transmitted through sex or there's no known cases and shit like that but . . . so we didn't use protection the very first time. And it was, you know we agreed, there was a mutual agreement right and I knew that he was with the same girl for the last six years and they broke up about 4 months ago. And I knew that I was clean because I was in jail for the last 4-1/2 month you know.* [31 year old–street/escort/bars]

Another woman spoke of trusting her current boyfriend and not using condoms with him, but not trusting her previous boyfriend to be disease free so insisting on a condom with him. As the following exchange reveals, trust of the current boyfriend is based on having known him for a long period of time, and the fact that he has been tested for STIs, whereas distrust of her previous boyfriend was related to his injection drug use.

> *Respondent: . . . he [current boyfriend] was one of my brother's best friends for 18, 20 years. So I knew him and I knew what he was about and I needed to see papers and stuff like that and he asked to see papers on me and . . .*
>
> *Interviewer: Papers meaning what?*
>
> *Respondent: That he didn't have HIV or any kind of serious diseases and he got his and I got mine and that's how we started.*
>
> *Interviewer: So was there any discussion of using condoms?*
>
> *Respondent: No, we didn't need condoms, you know. I knew he had nothing and he knew I had nothing so, you know we were clear there . . .*
>
> *Respondent: . . . there was one guy I was with for 6 years . . . and that was condom, condom, condoms with him.*

Interviewer: And why was that?

Respondent: . . . Cause I knew his history and I–also he used to shoot needles. . . . [31 year old–street/escort]

For the women who did use condoms early in the relationship and then terminated condom use after a period of time, non-condom use was conditional on the understanding that their partner did not have other private sexual partners. For many women, non-condom use was related to trusting that their partner was committed to the relationship and monogamous. The women were clearly aware that a partner with multiple sexual relationships represented a high-risk situation for them–and in many instances their children.

The first two years, the only way we'd go with no condoms was if we both go through the testing, the AIDS testing, the full, you know, first, then the six months, then the year then once more after that, because you know, I'm not going to take that risk. If ever, at a point in our relationship, that I even hear or I even think that you're having an affair behind my back, then it's over and I'll go with condoms because I'm not going to take that risk, you know? I have more to look out for besides me, if I get sick, who's going to raise my kids, you know, so I have to think that way. [34 year old–street]

DISCUSSION

Historically, enormous efforts have been made to control women's sexuality, from chastity belts to property laws (Scott & Jackson, 1996). The policing of women's sexuality, and the double standard, is perhaps most visible in the case of female sex trade workers as it is the women, not the (typically male) clients who are most highly stigmatized and who are under the greatest amount of surveillance (Scott & Jackson, 1996). In Canada, Shaver (1996) reports that women involved in the sex trade are more likely than clients to be charged with prostitution-related offences, and there is evidence that the charges against women in the sex trade are more severe than those against clients.

Davidson (1998) argues that although prostitution is popularly defined as the exchange of sex or sexual services for money and/or other material benefits, "it is better conceptualized as an institution which allows certain powers of command over one person's body to be exercised by another" (p.9). Many of the women we interviewed talked about the control clients have over the women especially in terms of abuse or the potential for abuse, but there was also a sense that the women had their own power, and were resistant to client control. In particular, when the women spoke of condom use their confidence in their ability to exert their will was evident in that they reported maintaining their insistence on condom use even, at times, when the client refused and even when doing so was potentially dangerous. Although the women provide a service that has been commodified, and do so in a context of few institutionalized supports (beyond community supports for sex trade workers) and much public disdain for what they do, many spoke of setting the conditions of the exchange, and doing so confidently especially in terms of condom use.

In some instances, the women spoke of the association of condoms with "professional" prostitutes and "clean prostitutes" juxtaposing this section of the population to "dirty," "unprofessional" prostitutes. The unprofessional sex trade workers were often linked to the drug-using women. A few of the women who reported using drugs indicated that they sometimes provide services without a condom although in most instances the women suggested that these services were low risk because of the type of service provided (e.g., oral sex) and/or because they believed the client was "clean." Still, in a few cases, the women reported providing higher risk sexual services (e.g., vaginal intercourse) without a condom, and this finding supports other researchers' suggestions that drug addicted women may be most susceptible to the nonuse of condoms (see, for example, Sterk, 1999; McDonnell, McDonnell, O'Neill & Mulcahy, 1998).

It is widely recognized that addictions, and especially periods of intense withdrawal, can cloud any "rational" thoughts and this may include practices related to condom use. Indeed, drug use may override the "agency" that many of our participants reported vis-à-vis condom use. The relationship between non-condom use and drug addiction is most likely a complex relationship, and future research is needed to unravel the ways in which women with different types and lengths of addiction, and under particular circumstances (e.g., great economic need) may be more or less susceptible to non-condom use. Further, although only one woman with a reported mental health problem indicated non-condom use, this may be a more significant problem than recognized to date, and research is needed to understand how best to address non-condom use among women with reported mental health problems and/or mental health and drug addiction issues.

A number of the women indicated that they were attempting to enter recovery programs but were having difficulties obtaining access, although since the completion of this study, a community-based low-threshold methadone programme has been established. The degree to which female sex trade workers who are entering the program might be better able to provide consistent condom use at work is a potential future research project. Still, our research does provide some level of optimism about condom use among drug using women given that a number of the women indicated that they always provided services with a condom. There is the possibility that they are simply indicating they use condoms because of what one woman suggested was the "shame" associated with non-condom use. However, given the multiple positive influences and forces encouraging condom use in this community these reports may be accurate.

In discussing female sex trade workers within the South African context, Campbell (2000) suggests that the women's life histories point to many factors that have minimized their sense of themselves as confident and valuable, and that this lack of confidence, in conjunction with the social organization of their home and working lives, and the social norms related to condom use, underline the relatively consistent nonuse of condoms while working. Campbell's account of the women's lives and the forces which led the women into the sex trade are strikingly similar to the stories told by many of the women we interviewed for the study reported on here. However, in the case of the women that we interviewed, there was, for many, great confidence in their ability to use condoms with clients, and this confidence appears to be situated within the context of their working lives and the relations into which they enter while working as well as the meanings attached to the use of condoms at work. Within this sex-trade community, there appears to be an acknowledgment of the importance of condoms, supported through relations with others such as escort service owners, other women involved in the sex trade and even some clients. This is not to say that resistance to condoms does not occur, or that all within the industry are supportive of condom use, or even that condoms are always utilized within the prostitute-client relationship. Rather, what we are suggesting is that there is a general culture of condom use that is reinforced and accepted through various relationships, and this culture appears to provide a valuable context supporting the women's confidence in their ability to maintain relatively consistent use of condoms with clients.

McKeganey et al. (1990) have noted, based on their work with female prostitutes in Glasgow, that women typically take a very "managerial" style at work, insisting upon condom use with clients. These researchers argue that one cannot overstate the degree to which the women have power vis-à-vis clients, but they do often have control over the condom use aspect of the encounter. Our work has found a similar pattern of "control" over the use of condoms with clients yet at times this "power" or "control" is expressed in a very covert manner as when the women feel they will not be able to convince the client about the importance of condom use so they surreptitiously put a condom on. The women are cognizant of the fact that in some instances it is dangerous to discuss or insist upon condom use, and they have learned alternative strategies for ensuring that they are protected, and this appears to add to their confidence vis-à-vis condom use.

In places where there is less consistent condom use with clients, as has been noted in the South African context (Campbell, 2000; Wojciki & Malala, 2001), much work may be needed to educate individuals who are part of the sex trade industry, beyond sex trade workers themselves, about the importance of condoms. The nature of relations outside the immediate prostitute-client relationship appears to play an important role in the consistent use of condoms within the prostitute-client relationship as it is such "external" relations that may provide additional supports for women's sense of confidence to insist on condom use. External supports and relations may also help to make clients cognizant of the importance of condoms thus creating less resistance on the part of clients and adding to the women's ability to use condoms.

The association of condoms with the health and safety of the women was a dominant theme in our study that appeared both to help reinforce the importance of condoms to the women themselves, and to assist them in their discussions with clients who were resistant to condom use. For a number of the women, health and safety went beyond their own personal concerns to include the health of their families. Condoms represent remaining healthy to continue to work to support economically not only themselves but also family members, especially children. Many of the women spoke of entering the sex trade industry in order to obtain needed economic resources, and therefore, it is not surprising that the emphasis placed on remaining healthy was linked to their role as breadwinner for their family. However, to date, many prevention programmes have not recognized the importance of the women's private lives, and especially their roles of mother and "breadwinner," in motivating them to use condoms at work–as well as at home. Women have been abstracted from their everyday lives, yet it is in the context of their lives and their relationships with children and families that we may find one of the greatest motivators to condom use.

Within the HIV discourse on prostitution, women involved in the sex trade are typically viewed as "workers," and there is relatively little discussion of other aspects of their lives particularly their roles of mother and wife. In part this is because of the women's own resistance to discussing their private lives given the potential negative repercussions for their family and/or themselves. However, in places where there continues to be nonuse of condoms among female sex trade workers, prevention programs should find strategies to emphasize the women's private lives, and the importance of staying healthy for their own good and the good of their family/children.

Although many of the women we interviewed reported relatively consistent condom use with clients, the pattern was quite the opposite when they discussed condom use with private partners, and this is a dichotomy that others have found (McKeganey & Barnard, 1992, Pyett & Warr, 1997). For at least some of the women, the private sphere is the place where one seeks comfort and safety from the day-to-day problems and challenges of work. Many of the women define sexual relations at "home" as pleasurable and representing a source of love and commitment, symbolized through the nonuse of condoms. At the same time, however, some of the women spoke of the violence within their private relations pointing to the pain of private relations. As many feminists have noted, the discourse of the home as a haven in a heartless world does not match the experience of many women, and gender relations in the home can be at one and the same time both pleasurable and a source of pain (Scott & Jackson, 1996).

In some instances, the woman's lack of power in the relationship or the partner's dislike of condoms and the association of condoms with the sex trade appear to be key reasons for the nonuse of condoms with private partners. But as noted above, in many instances the women also play a key role in the decision not to use a condom and condoms are a "sometimes" practice. It is not that all the women are without agency in their private relations and are simply playing the "traditional" role of the passive woman providing sexual services to their "man" without the use of protection. Nor is it that they are unaware of risks associated with sexual relations at home as some of the women's accounts point to concerns about their health and well-being vis-à-vis STIs including HIV. Indeed, the nonuse of condoms should not be interpreted as a lack of knowledge about risks or a disinterest in risk management. Rather, it appears that a number of the women utilize different strategies within the context of their private relations to ensure their safety, including using a condom during the early period of the relationship until they and their partner are tested for various diseases, insisting upon monogamy within their private relationship, and/or demanding honesty of their partner so that condoms can be used if their partner has other relationships.

This research suggests that for many of the women there is not a strong belief in the need to use condoms with private partners at least in part because other means of ensuring safety (such as being tested for STIs) are available and can be utilized. In other locations where testing is not available, and in particular in many Third World countries, such a strategy is probably not an option although in some contexts the women may be utilizing different strategies that future research will need to uncover. Many of the women we spoke to were well aware that there was the potential for contracting STIs including HIV from a private partner but given that they were not interested in using condoms and/or their partner was not interested/resisted use (in part because of the association of condoms with work) other techniques were utilized for protecting their health. From a public health point of view such strategies might be viewed as creating limited and contingent protection, but they do point to the fact that the women are knowledgeable of the risks of HIV within the private setting. It appears that it is not that the women deny risks of infection within their private lives, but rather, that the condom does not "fit" within the context of their private lives, and other methods of reducing risks–or at least the belief that they are reducing risks–are utilized as the women are active agents in protecting their health.

Findings from this study support the notion that condom use is related to the specific socio-cultural context within which women live and work, and that there are constraints and opportunities for condom use within certain settings. For the female sex trade workers in this community, responses to risks and risk management have taken on different forms within the public and private spheres, creating variable times and contexts for condom use. For many of the women we spoke to, condoms with clients appear to be an accepted part of the sex trade culture, and it is the non-use of condoms that is viewed as outside of the norm. At the same time, within the context of the women's private relations condoms are used consistently for some, not at all for others, and for many women they are part of an overall strategy to reduce risks, and as part of this strategy they are used only under certain conditions and "sometimes." Although as feminist works have noted, the balance of power in heterosexual relationships together with cultural discourses and sexual scripts, may militate against women negotiating safer sex, at least some of the women in this study have developed strategies for creating for themselves safer sexual relations, albeit contingent safety (Scott & Jackson, 1996).

REFERENCES

Alexander, P. (1997). Feminism, sex workers and human rights. In J. Nagle (Ed.), *Whores and other feminists* (pp.83-97). New York: Routledge.

Barnard, M. (1993). Violence and vulnerability: conditions of work for streetworking prostitutes. *Sociology of Health and Illness, 5,* 683-705.

Campbell, C. (2000). Selling sex in the time of AIDS: the psycho-social context of condom use by sex workers on a Southern African mine. *Social Science & Medicine, 50* (4), 479-494.

Dalla, R. (2000). Exposing the "pretty woman" myth: a qualitative examination of the lives of female streetwalking prostitutes. *The Journal of Sex Research, 37*(4), 344-353.

Davidson, J. (1998). *Prostitution, power and freedom.* Ann Arbor: University of Michigan Press.

Donegan, C. (1996). Prostitutes can help prevent the transmission of HIV. *Nursing Times, 92,* 38-39.

Dorfman, L., Derish, P., & Cohen, J. (1992). Hey girlfriend: an evaluation of AIDS prevention among women in the sex industry. *Health Education Quarterly, 19*(1), 25-40.

Erickson, P., Butters, J., McGillicuddy, P., & Hallgren, A. (2000). Crack and prostitution: gender, myths and experiences. *Journal of Drug Issues, 30* (4), 767-788.

Gavey, N., McPhillips, K., & Doherty, M. (2001). If It's Not On, It's Not On–Or Is It? Discursive Constraints on Women's Condom Use. *Gender and Society, 15*:917-43.

Green, S.T., Goldberg, D.J., Christie, P.R., Frischer, M., Thomson, A., Carr, S.V., et al. (1993). Female prostitutes in Glasgow: a descriptive study of their lifestyle. *AIDS Care, 5*(3), 321-335.

Jackson, L., Highcrest, A., & Coates, R. (1992). Varied potential risks of HIV infection among female prostitutes. *Social Science and Medicine, 35* (3), 281-286.

Jackson, L. & Hood, C. (2001). Men's leisure, women's work: Female prostitutes and the double standard of North American HIV public health policies. In J. Anderson & L. Lawrence (Eds.), *Gender Issues in Work and Leisure* (pp.29 37). Eastbourne: Leisure Studies Association.

Scott, S., & Jackson, S. (1996). Sexual Skirmishes and Feminist Factions: Twenty-five Years of Debate on Women and Sexuality. In S. Jackson & S. Scott, (Eds.), *Feminism and Sexuality: A Reader* (1-31). New York: Columbia University Press.

Jesson, J., Luck, M., & Taylor, J. (1994). Working women in the sex industry and their perception of risk from HIV/AIDS. *Health Care for Women International, 15*(1): 3-9.

Kinnell, H. (1991). Prostitutes' perceptions of risk and factors related to risk-taking. In P. Aggleton, G. Hart, & P. Davies (Eds.), *AIDS: Responses, interventions and care* (pp. 79-94). London: Farmer Press.

Liam, W., Chan, R., & Wee, S. (2000). Sex workers' perspectives on condom use for oral sex with clients: a qualitative study. *Health Education Behaviour, 27*(4): 502-516.

Maticka-Tyndale, E. & Lewis, J. (1999). *Escort services in a border town: Transmission dynamics of sexually transmitted infections within and between communities.* Health Canada Report. Ottawa: Division of STD Prevention and Control, Laboratory Centres for Disease Control.

McDonnell, R., McDonnell, P., O'Neill, M., & Mulcahy, F. (1998). Health risk profile of prostitutes in Dublin. *International Journal of STDs and AIDS, 9.*, 485-488.

McKeganey, N, Barnard, M., & Bloor, M. (1990). A comparison of HIV-related risk behaviour and risk reduction between female street working prostitutes and male rent boys in Glasgow. *Sociology of Health & Illness, 12*(3), 274-292.

McKeganey, N., & Barnard, M. (1992). *AIDS, drugs and sexual risk: lives in the balance.* Philadelphia: Open University Press.

McLeod, E. (1982). *Working women: Prostitution now.* London: Croom Helm.

Pyett, P., & Warr, D. (1997). Vulnerability on the streets: Female sex workers and HIV risk. *AIDS Care* 9(5), 539-547.

Scambler, G., Peswani, R., Renton, A. & Scambler, A. (1990). Women prostitutes in the AIDS era. *Sociology of Health & Illness, 2*(3), 260-273.

Scott, S. & Jackson, S. (1996). Sexual Skirmishes and Feminist Factions: Twenty-five years of debate on women and sexuality. In S. Jackson & S. Scott (Eds.), Feminism and Sexuality. New York: Columbia University Press.

Shaver, F. (1996). The regulation of prostitution: Setting the morality trap. In B. Schissel & L. Mahood (Eds.), *Social control in Canada: A reader on the social construction of deviance.* (pp.204-226). Toronto: Oxford University Press.

Sterk, C. (1999). *Fast lives: Women who use crack cocaine.* Philadelphia: Temple University Press.

Strauss, A. (1987) *Qualitative analysis for social scientists.* Cambridge: Cambridge University Press.

Surratt, H., Wechsberg, W., Cottler, L., & Leukefeld, C. (1998). Acceptability of the female condom among women at risk for HIV infection. *The American Behavioural Scientist, 41*(8), 1157-1170.

Vanwesenbeeck, I., van Zessen, G., De Graaf, R. & Straver, C. (1994). Contextual and interactional factors influencing condom use in heterosexual prostitution contacts. *Patient Education and Counseling, 24*, 307-322.

Venema, P. & Visser, J. (1990). Safer prostitution: a new approach in Holland. In M. Plant (Ed.), *AIDS, drugs and prostitution* (pp.41-60). London: Routledge.

Weiner, A. (1996). Understanding the social needs of streetwalking prostitutes. *Social Work, 41*(1), 97-105.

Wojciki, J. & Malala, J. (2001). Condom use, power and HIV/AIDS risk: sex workers bargain for survival in Hilbrow/Joubert Part/Berea, Johannesburg. *Social Science & Medicine, 53*(1), 99-121.

Youth Services Bureau. (1991). *Ottawa Street Prostitutes: A Survey.* Unpublished document. Ottawa.

Racial and Ethnic Segmentation of Female Prostitution in Los Angeles County

Janet Lever, PhD
David E. Kanouse, PhD
Sandra H. Berry, PhD

SUMMARY. Previous studies of female sex workers engaged in prostitution have focused primarily on street-based workers, who are more visible and approachable than women working off the street. As part of a study estimating the size and characteristics of the work force of female prostitutes in Los Angeles County, we examined the hidden population of women who solicit clients in private locales off the street. Data sources included law enforcement personnel and staff in other government agencies; ethnographic informants; directories and other written materials; and the World Wide Web. Results show a high degree of ra-

---

Janet Lever is Professor of Sociology at California State University at Los Angeles. David E. Kanouse and Sandra H. Berry are Senior Behavioral Scientists at the RAND Corporation, Santa Monica, CA.

Address correspondence to: David E. Kanouse, The RAND Corporation, 1776 Main Street, Santa Monica, CA 90407 (E-mail: kanouse@rand.org).

This research was supported by grants R01HD24897 from the Demographic and Behavioral Sciences Branch, National Institute of Child Health and Human Development, and P30MH058107 from the National Institute of Mental Health. The authors thank Diane Gurman, Rosanna Hertz, and R. Stephen Warner for helpful comments on a draft.

[Haworth co-indexing entry note]: "Racial and Ethnic Segmentation of Female Prostitution in Los Angeles County." Lever, Janet, David E. Kanouse, and Sandra H. Berry. Co-published simultaneously in *Journal of Psychology & Human Sexuality* (The Haworth Press, Inc.) Vol. 17, No. 1/2, 2005, pp. 107-129; and: *Contemporary Research on Sex Work* (ed: Jeffrey T. Parsons) The Haworth Press, Inc., 2005, pp. 107-129. Single or multiple copies of this article are available for a fee from The Haworth Document Delivery Service [1-800-HAWORTH, 9:00 a.m. - 5:00 p.m. (EST). E-mail address: docdelivery@haworthpress.com].

Digital Object Identifier: 10.1300/J056v17n01_07   *107*

cial and ethnic segmentation in the sex industry, reflecting an influx of
ethnic entrepreneurs who market prostitution in culturally specific ways.
[Article copies available for a fee from The Haworth Document Delivery Ser-
vice: *1-800-HAWORTH. E-mail address: <docdelivery@haworthpress.com>
Website: <http://www.HaworthPress.com>* © 2005 by The Haworth Press, Inc.
All rights reserved.]*

KEYWORDS. Female sex workers, prostitution, racial and ethnic differences, solicitation venues

Empirical research on female sex workers in the past 20 years has focused mainly on street prostitutes, the most visible segment of the sex
worker population. Less is known about women who solicit clients in
other locales, by advertising their services or through referral networks.
Yet, a great deal of commercial sex activity in most communities in the
U.S. occurs off the street, in massage parlors, clubs, brothels, and other
private locales. This paper draws on data collected on female sex
workers in Los Angeles (LA) County.

In the last four decades, LA has become one of the most racially and
ethnically diverse cities of the world. The LA Almanac (2004) indicates
that from 1960-2000, foreign-born residents increased from 8% to 36%,
a net gain of 3.8 million. The 2000 census showed that Latinos replaced
Whites as the largest ethnic group (44.6% vs. 31.1%), and Asian-Amer-
icans displaced African-Americans as the third largest racial/ethnic
group (11.8% vs. 9.5%).

This enormous influx of immigrants has transformed the labor market. Entrepreneurship, including illegal enterprise, has long been recognized as an important survival and mobility strategy for immigrant and
minority groups (Fischer & Massey, 2000). Ethnic entrepreneurs often
find market opportunities serving the needs and preferences of their
own community. This is likely to be true for sexual needs and preferences as well–especially if the social context surrounding commercial
sex in the immigrant subculture differs from that found in the dominant
culture. Light (1977) contrasted the participation of African Americans
and Chinese in prostitution, the largest part of the vice industry, from
1880 to 1944 in American industrial cities. African American women
were streetwalkers, while Chinese women worked out of syndicated
brothels, leading to the conclusion that socio-cultural characteristics are
as important as supply and demand in determining how illegal services
are marketed.

For some, prostitution is an occupation of economic desperation, chosen because it offers the best option for meeting survival goals and/or supporting a drug habit. In LA, African American and Latina women are overrepresented at the bottom of the economic ladder. Low-income sex workers often work on the streets, where entry barriers are low but vulnerability to violence and arrest is high. In LA, we would expect such women to be predominantly African American or Latina because Whites and Asian Americans enjoy greater economic advantages.

Differences in types of prostitutes have been noted in previous research. Jackson, Highcrest, and Coates (1992) distinguished three types: street prostitutes, escorts, and those who work as part-time prostitutes within the service sector (e.g., erotic massage therapists). However, these three types are not exhaustive; for example, full-time brothel workers are excluded. Winick and Kinsie (1971), drawing on over 2,000 interviews with prostitutes, clients, and other informants, provided a remarkably comprehensive description of the various ways in which female sex workers in the U.S. plied their trade from the 1930s through the 1960s. Although new forms have emerged since then, we have used an approach similar to theirs by describing market segments based on how and where prostitutes solicit clients. There are three basic methods by which prostitutes make their availability known to clients: (1) being present in a location where clients will either notice them or expect to find them; (2) advertising their availability in a medium; and (3) through referral. The first two methods can be further subdivided according to the specific type of location or advertising. Among locations, it is useful to distinguish street from off-street locations, with further subdivisions among different types of off-street locations. For advertising, one can distinguish according to what types of services are advertised (e.g., outcall massage, escorts) and/or in what media (e.g., yellow pages, sex tabloids, Internet). Sex workers who obtain clients only through referrals are known as call girls.

Studies of female street prostitutes in the U.S. tend to fall into two categories: (1) intensive interviews with small convenience samples of women, exploring selected topics related to sex work, drug use, or experience with violence victimization (Freund, Leonard & Lee, 1989; Romero-Daza et al., 2003; Witte, Wada, El-Bassel, Gilbert, & Wallace, 2000); and (2) larger, quantitative studies focusing on HIV-related risk behavior and/or HIV or Hepatitis B serostatus, which have recruited women through outreach efforts or from STI clinics, jails or detention centers (Rosenblum et al., 1992; Suratt & Inciardi, 2004) or identified them from larger samples of drug users (Jones et al., 1998; Paone, Cooper, Alperen, Shi, & Des Jarlais, 1999). These samples tend to include mostly women from the street-based segment of the population. In nearly all of these studies that have been conducted in large cities, a majority of the women are racial or ethnic minorities, with African Americans most heavily represented. The same has been true in medium-sized Eastern cities such as Camden (Freund, Leonard, & Lee, 1989) and Hartford (Romero-Daza et al., 2003). Racial and ethnic minorities have been less dominant in samples of female sex workers from medium-sized cities in the Midwest (Williamson & Folaron, 2001), South (Kuhns, Heide, & Silverman, 1992), and West (Bellis, 1990; Potterat et al., 2004).

In general, previous research has found that off-street female sex workers tend to be predominantly White in the advertising and referral strata (Seidlin et al., 1988), and either White, Asian, or Latina in the lo-cale-based strata. Seventy percent of workers in two legal brothels in Nevada interviewed in 1995 were White (Albert, Warner, & Hatcher, 1998). In contrast, Deren and colleagues (1996) studied Dominican prostitutes in New York City who worked in brothels or on the street, finding that women working on the street were more acculturated. A re-cent study of women working in massage parlors in San Francisco found that 81% of those interviewed were Vietnamese (Nemoto, Operario, Takenaka, Iwamoto, & Le, 2003).

Hong and Duff (1997) studied taxi-dance clubs in LA during the mid-1990s, and reported that in clubs catering to Latino men, the host-esses were Latina, but in clubs that served an Asian or mixed clientele, the hostesses were mostly White; in the more recently emerged ta-ble-dance clubs, most dancers were White. Thompson and Harred (1992) interviewed topless dancers from six clubs in a major city in the Southwest, many of whom also performed personalized table dances, and 82% of these dancers were White.

The goal of this study is to describe the racial/ethnic representation of prostitution among different types of female sex workers in LA County, including street prostitutes, women that clients find in off-street locales, and women whom clients find via advertised phone numbers, Internet links, or personal referral from madams or other clients.

METHODS

Beginning in 1990, we conducted a community-wide study of female sex workers in LA County, with the goal of describing the workforce of women engaged in prostitution (i.e., who accepted payments for specific acts involving masturbation or oral, vaginal, or anal sex with their clients). We conducted interviews with women working on and off the street. We also interviewed ethnographic informants, conducted archival research in directories and other documents, and examined advertising in newspapers and on the World Wide Web.

Participants and Procedures

Elsewhere we describe the methods we used to construct a spatial-temporal sampling frame to recruit a probability sample of female street prostitutes in the 4,000 square mile area of LA County (Kanouse et al., 1999). Field staff randomly selected women on the street, screened them for study eligibility, conducted interviews, and took blood samples.

The bulk of our data about off-street prostitution came from interviews and written materials collected and analyzed between July 1989 and December 1991. Updated information was solicited in 1996 and again in 2003-2004. Table 1 summarizes the sources of data available for each of the four strata of female sex workers. Having multiple sources allowed us to examine consistency of data across sources. Most data presented in this paper were obtained from ethnographic informants and government agencies with a "need to know." For greater detail, especially on our use of written reports, records, and documents, see Lever and Kanouse (1998). In addition, in the early years of the study, White male and female field investigators visited massage parlors, and went on "ride-alongs" with divisional vice officers, while a Korean male investigated Asian clubs, hotels, and massage parlors.

Information was collected from policing agencies in two ways. First, staff conducted structured interviews with an officer in the vice squad of the 18 precincts of the LA Police Department (LAPD), 37 detective bureaus of the independent municipalities, and 17 stations of the County Sheriff's Department. Although the focus of these interviews was to determine the precise locations and times of day and night for street prostitution, each interviewee was also asked if there were "motels, sex shops, sex bookstores, bars, topless clubs, massage parlors, etc." where prostitution occurred in their community, followed by another item that asked about tourist and business hotels. Unstructured interviews were conducted by senior staff with several representatives of Organized Crime and Vice, the citywide arm of LAPD, which is responsible for policing prostitution "above the streets"; two detectives on its Asian

TABLE 1. Principal Sources of Information About Female Prostitution in Los Angeles County

Strata	Sources	Dominant Race/Ethnicity of Sex Workers
I. Streetwalkers	Vice squads in 18 precincts of LAPD	African-American
	Detective bureaus in 37 independent municipalities	
	Vice departments in 17 stations of Sheriff's Department	
	23 health districts of LA County Dept. of Health Services	
	Pasadena and Long Beach Health Services	
	Informants (health educators and outreach workers)	
II. Advertisement (escorts)	LAPD, esp. citywide Vice and Hollywood precinct	White, Non-Hispanic
	Sheriff's Vice Division	
	District and City Attorneys	
	Yellow Pages (under "escort" and "massage")	
	Sex tabloids and alternative press	
	Informants (owners, managers, dispatcher)	
	Off-street sex worker interviews	
III. Referral-Based (call girls)	LAPD, citywide Vice Division	White, Non-Hispanic
	Hollywood precinct, LAPD	
	Beverly Hills Police Dept.	
	District Attorney's Office	
	Madams (10+ women in "stable")	
	Mini-madams (under 10 women in "stable")	
IV. Locale-Based Massage parlor workers (on premises)	Commission Investigation Division, LAPD	Asian
	Sheriff, Vice Division	
	Asian Task Force	
	City clerk tax and permit system	
	Yellow Pages listings	
	Informants (owner, fieldworkers)	
	Newport Beach and San Diego Vice Detectives	

Strata	Sources	Dominant Race/Ethnicity of Sex Workers
Hotels–Class A	L.A. Convention and Visitors Bureau membership list (City and County) Fire Dept. Assemblage Control Division LAPD Administrative and Divisional Vice Municipalities' Detective Bureaus Sheriff, Vice Division Informants (former and current hotel employees, escorts, and field workers)	White, Non-Hispanic
Adult Cabaret a. Clubs featuring nudity b. Gambling clubs	Alcoholic Beverage Control County Tax Collector City Zoning and Building and Safety Sheriff, Vice Division Hollywood Precinct, LAPD Informants (cultural consultants, fieldworkers)	White, Non-Hispanic
Asian Hostess Clubs	Alcoholic Beverage Control State Labor Board LAPD Asian Task Force and Vice Sheriff, Vice Division Korean Cafe and Nightclub Association Informants (cultural consultants, fieldworkers)	Asian
Bars a. Cantinas (for new Hispanic immigrants) b. Neighborhood bars	Alcoholic Beverage Control State Labor Board Immigration and Naturalization Services LAPD Divisional Vice Municipalities' Detective Bureaus Sheriff, Vice STD field investigators Informants (fieldworkers, outreach specialists)	Hispanic Immigrant
Brothels	LAPD and Sheriff, Administrative Vice Informants (madams)	Asian
Hostess Dance Halls (Taxi-dance)	Alcoholic Beverage Control LAPD, Precinct-Level Vice Squad Informants (dancers, academic researchers, filmmaker)	Hispanic Immigrant, White

Detail of Organized Crime (specialists in Japanese and Korean cultures); one from the Special Investigations Bureau, and two consecutive heads of the Commission Investigation Division, which oversees the city's massage parlors and grants permits to incall and outcall massage technicians. Their counterparts in the Sheriff's headquarters were interviewed, as were specialists in the Hollywood Division of LAPD and the Beverly Hills Police Department's vice squad. Most in-depth information was collected between 1989-1991; shorter interviews in 2003-2004 focused on changes noted, and reasons for them, in off-street prostitution over the duration of our study. Sources from the judicial sector of law enforcement are noted in Table 1.

Similar structured and unstructured interviews were conducted in 1989-1990 with representatives of all districts of the Department of Health Services (DHS), including high-ranking staff within the Disease Control Program and the AIDS Program. Selected representatives in the regional offices of DHS were interviewed for updates in 2003-2004. Representatives of all five regional offices of the Alcoholic Beverage Control (ABC) were interviewed in both 1989-1991 and 2003-2004. All 998 street sex workers who were interviewed in the first years of the study were asked to name off-street locations that they associated with prostitution, and their information confirmed what was learned from other sources.

Other government agencies that provided information are noted in Table 1, as is the broad category "ethnographic informants." The latter can be divided into several subcategories: 13 academic researchers, nine outreach practitioners with expertise and contacts in various strata of prostitution (including cantinas), nine persons with expertise in related occupations (e.g., ad-takers in sex tabloids, lawyers well-known for representing massage parlor owners or madams, and a telephone operator who worked with two escort agencies), and 16 current and past sex worker informants (e.g., support group facilitators, labor organizers, madams, owners of escort agencies and massage parlors, and taxi dancers). All informants were interviewed in the early years of the study; a few were re-interviewed for updated information in 1996 and 2003-2004.

The content of the unstructured interviews focused, where appropriate, on what the interviewee knew about off-street prostitution in LA County and on what basis (e.g., undercover surveillance); the modus operandi for attracting customers and evading law enforcement; the age, race/ethnicity, and citizenship of the sex workers and clientele; sexual acts, including price and sexual risk-taking; the percentage of women on the premises actually involved in the sex trade; whether any also ever work on the streets; and, finally, whether there were any records that we could review to learn more. As a further source of information on off-street prostitution, we conducted interviews with 83 women who worked primarily in the advertising and referral strata, recruited via a mass media campaign, ads in the popular press and sex tabloids, cold-calling of their advertised numbers, and by referral from previous participants.

Also, we followed relevant stories in the *Los Angeles Times* for over a decade; for example, a series of articles reporting a lap-dance ban (Garrison, 2003a; 2003b) and subsequent repeal by the LA City Council (Garrison, 2003b) provided valuable information about the number of adult clubs in the city and the rules governing dancer/customer interactions. By the mid-1990s, an additional valuable source of information became available: the World Wide Web. For example, WorldSexGuide.org and citigirls.com have local guides where male clients can share information on which establishments provide sexual services, how to get past their front of legitimacy, which women to ask for, and prices. Google searches using the keywords "escorts Los Angeles" yield thousands of sites that include women's photos and their ethnicity/race. These sources helped to update earlier information on aspects of local off-street prostitution.

RESULTS

Street Prostitutes

We completed 998 interviews with a probability sample of street prostitutes. Based on participants' self-reports, 69% of the 998 participants were African American, 17% White, 9% Hispanic, less than 1% Asian, and 4% mixed or other.

Advertising and Referral

Multiple sources of data show that the women who worked through escort services and those who worked through referral networks (mostly through madams and mini-madams) were predominantly White. There was remarkable consistency between reports from the madams and a citywide vice detective who was widely reputed to know more about madams and call girls than anyone else. This detective, who had worked the prostitution detail for 20 years, provided us with numerical estimates for the uppermost tier of what he called "high-line call girls," estimates corroborated by LA's most famous madam at the time, Alex Adams, in an interview given to the *Los Angeles Times* in 1992 (Lait & Hubler, 1999).

We drew on this detective's "four-tiered pyramid of players" and the ethnic/racial composition of the "stables" of women workers as the most reliable source of information available. Countywide there were seven madams for high-end services and about 20 "major madams" in the top two tiers, meaning madams who had exclusive access to 10 to 20 call girls at a time. The call girls were 20 to 25 years old in the top tier, a little older in the second tier, and all of them were White. He told us that if a madam gets a request for an African American or Asian woman, she would know whom to call, but they would not be part of her regular stable, and there were not many such requests. Operations in the two lower tiers were run by women he called "mini-madams," who could call on five or six women in their late 20s to early 30s. He estimated that there were about 200 mini-madams in the county at the beginning of our study, of whom about 85% were White, 10% African American, 4% Asian, and no more than 1% Latina.

Women who worked in advertised escort or dating services were also predominantly White. One owner of a service advertised in several major Yellow Pages directories told us that she had 15 to 20 White women she could call on, and that she knew one Asian woman, but she would not include her among her "regulars." She said that she made contacts with four African-American women but never succeeded in getting work for them. Two others who had managed escort services for many years said the same. Another informant, a telephone dispatcher for two widely advertised escort services, said that she had contact information on about 50 escorts who were mostly White, but included 8 African American, 4 Hispanic, and 2 Asian women. One of our escort informants who had worked for many agencies for over a decade said that in all that time, she had only met 2 African American women, 1 Asian woman, and no Latina women. Examination of the photos and profiles of women on Los Angeles escort service Web sites supported the conclusion that this stratum was still predominantly White, although the proportion of Latina women appears to have grown since our study began.

Locale-Based Prostitution

Massage Parlors. Massage parlors are so closely associated with prostitution that businesses offering strictly therapeutic massage include terms like "legitimate" or "nonsexual" in their advertisements. We approached a dozen Korean-run parlors that were under surveillance by LAPD, but we were unable to get past the manager to reach either owners or workers. Police records indicate that in raids they catch customers engaging in oral and vaginal intercourse, sometimes without a condom. They have confiscated canisters with 100-200 condoms, which are later used as evidence of illegal activity, further discouraging condom use.

As of 2004, the LAPD's monitoring for prostitution was focused on 25 licensed massage parlors and 25 acupressure and aromatherapy centers that circumvented the permit and zoning requirements for licensed parlors. Vice personnel from both LAPD and the Sheriff's Department told us that the latest "front" to evade police regulation was to run prostitution rings through chiropractors' clinics. A recent *Los Angeles Times* article explained the change (Morin, 2002). Unlike acupressure clinics, chiropractors are allowed to feature massage, and their assistants require no licensing. California chiropractors, desperate for revenue as their ranks keep growing while insurance reimbursements shrink, get lured by ads and approached by "business managers" who offer to provide a variety of massage therapists to boost income. The number of massage establishments varied as police surveillance changed over time, based on budgets and other priorities. After their growth spurt in the 1970s, from the early 1980s to the mid-1990s, the number of massage parlors declined dramatically in LA, as in other major cities. About 50 licensed parlors were under surveillance for prostitution then. Many massage businesses merely moved from the city into unincorporated parts of the county or into the small municipalities without the resources for undercover police; others moved further into Orange and Ventura Counties because of their more lenient licensing requirements.

In our 2003-2004 update, we learned that prostitution locations featuring massage had grown substantially, in large part due to the movement to unregulated venues that are more difficult to monitor. Combining conservative estimates from LAPD and the Sheriff's expert on prostitution, there are at least 200 businesses throughout LA County. This includes licensed massage parlors, chiropractic and acupressure clinics, and skin and tanning salons.

Another reason for growth is that Asian immigrants arrived in large numbers from countries with long-established red light districts that produced a climate of expectation and acceptance for patronage of prostitutes (Allison, 1994; Truong, 1990). Because of the many Asian ethnic groups, law enforcement lacks agents with the language skills needed for undercover work in the unregulated clinic sites. Moreover, Internet sites and proliferating foreign-language newspapers successfully expand the client base for adult businesses. In LA County, another reason for growth was the severe cutback in the number of officers assigned to vice detail, from 24 at the beginning of our study to 4 in 2004. Because each of the 18 LAPD precincts has its own vice squad, law enforcement in the city has been more constant.

Another significant change since our study began involves the ethnic backgrounds of the masseuses. Customers are as diverse as the area's population, but in the licensed parlors of LA County, Koreans have held a near monopoly as owners and technicians. Many women live on the premises and are barely conversant in English. In the unlicensed businesses that offer massage services, the situation has changed dramatically in recent years. There is typically a "mama-san" (host/manager) who is Asian, but vice experts estimate that up to half of the masseuses who work in unregulated venues in the city are now immigrant Latinas. In the County, by contrast, most unregulated businesses featuring massage are run by Chinese entrepreneurs and use Chinese immigrant women almost exclusively.

Nightclubs. The term "nightclub" covers many types of entertainment establishments, ranging from neighborhood bars to exclusive clubs with expensive cover charges. Whereas one might think that prostitution can be found in all types, we found only a limited number were involved in the sex trade, and that they were highly segmented by race/ethnicity. Mostly White women, and a few African American and Latina women, were found working in clubs featuring nudity. We did not hear of any casual neighborhood bars catering to White or African American clientele that were associated routinely with prostitution; perhaps this vacuum is due to the easy availability of African American sex workers on the streets and White women via the many modes of advertisement. By contrast, neighborhood bars for Latino immigrants were regularly monitored by the ABC for illegal activities, including prostitution. Asian nightclubs, whether catering to a middle-class or wealthy clientele, are also known to insiders as places were "hostesses" sometimes provide more than companionship.

- *Adult Cabarets and Other Establishments with Nudity.* Many suspect that adult cabarets featuring nudity are fronts for organized prostitution. But only occasionally did our informants provide any hint that cabaret owners were involved in prostitution in contemporary LA. Their businesses were described as very lucrative and the alcohol license as too precious to risk losing on account of a prostitution charge. Nevertheless, customers and dancers acknowledged that occasionally "hand jobs," oral sex, and even intercourse take place in darkened corners and VIP rooms. We assume that most dancers, waitresses, and bartenders who engage in prostitution do so discreetly on a freelance basis, without the participation of management.

There are 45 adult cabarets in LA and more than 50 such places scattered throughout the rest of the county. Smaller clubs feature about 5 women, while larger ones, like those near LA International Airport, may feature 10 to 15 women. Most of the dancers are young White women, and the great majority of customers are White as well. We heard of only five clubs where the dancers were mostly African American.

• *Asian Nightclubs.* The most common type of Asian nightclub is the "hostess bar," and according to the ABC, there are over 200 of them in Southern California, mostly clustered in Little Tokyo, Koreatown, Torrance, and Garden Grove, or scattered throughout the San Gabriel Valley, to serve both local and visiting Japanese, Korean, and Chinese businessmen (Braun, 1989). Their roots go back to the 1920s in Japan, when they were created as an inexpensive alternative to Japan's famous Geisha houses, and they have been thriving there ever since. Recreated here in the mid-1980s to carry on the cultural tradition, some hostess bars incorporated the modern "karaoke" machine or disco into the entertainment. Busy clubs have about 20 hostesses available to bring hot towels to a customer, talk to him, and laugh at his jokes. As in Tokyo and Hong Kong, fees for the hostess's time are folded into an unitemized bill where one hour may cost $300. As in much of Asia, where hostess clubs are an established part of entertaining clients (Allison, 1994), the bill is charged to an expense account.

Most customers cannot obtain more than teasing and "ritualized flirtation," part of a hostess' duties, making it difficult for police and the ABC. Actual sex for money is restricted to the elite–the richest customers–in the fancy Japanese clubs of Little Tokyo, more accessible to the upper middle-class in Koreatown clubs, and most widely available in the Chinese clubs.

Hostesses were also available in another type of Asian club where prostitution likely occurs. In one ABC district with a heavy concentration of Asians, investigators told us about immigrant

Asian women who work as hostesses and prostitutes in the 100 or so underground gambling clubs that have neither a gaming nor a liquor license. These clubs feature high-stakes games of Mahjong and Pai Gow poker, popular types of gambling among many Asians. Six card clubs in the LA area are large enough to be called casinos. Women play alongside men in these legal clubs and are not associated with prostitution. The underground clubs, however, are more like male preserves and believed to feature prostitution on their unregulated premises.

- *Cantinas.* "Cantina," like the saloons found all over Central America, is the name for bars catering to recent immigrants from Mexico and Central America. Only Spanish is spoken, and American-born Latinos say they look and feel as out of place in cantinas as "Anglos." They are not places a man would take a wife or girlfriend. The women here have what are described as "sullied reputations." A cantina without bar girls (B-girls) would be as inconceivable as one without liquor. Even the bartenders are mostly female to add to the allure for men.

It is a Central American tradition that men can find female companionship for drinking, talking, and dancing at a cantina, and they expect to pay more for a companion's drinks than for their own. The B-girl, who is not officially an employee and earns no wages, gets a kickback of $1-$7 per drink. Vice officers from 11 precincts told us that there is prostitution in cantinas in their districts; often the ABC is called in by police to investigate. Health department workers in several branch offices confirmed that some of their "index cases" (the client who presents symptoms at an STI clinic) name B-girls whom they met in cantinas as the likely source for their syphilis or gonorrhea. Researchers and outreach workers concerned with the spread of HIV within the Latino communities also recognize the health risks taken and posed by sex workers in the cantinas, where they estimate as many as 50% of B-girls are involved in prostitution

There are about 25 licensed large cantinas and 480 small ones, according to pooled estimates of the five ABC district offices. While agents for one ABC district estimated at least another 100 cantinas operating illegally, agents from the other four districts said that unlicensed places are quickly shut down in their areas. On average, small cantinas have at least 4 to 8 B-girls, with 10 or more working on a busy weekend night; large cantinas (each community with a sizeable Latino population has at least one large cantina) feature about 40 women on weekends. The women range in age from 18 to 40s (as many as 30% of the undocumented are believed to be under the legal drinking age), and the average age is about 27. The cantina B-girls are virtually all from Mexico and Central America, and an estimated 95% are undocumented. Sadly, some are trapped as "indentured servants," owing either the cantina owner or a "coyote" (a guide who helps undocumented immigrants cross the border) the $1,500 fee for bringing them into the U.S. Most often they were brought in by the cantina owner, who sets up all his new arrivals in the same apartment and expects sexual favors himself for giving them entry and a job.

Brothels and Other Private Places. At the start of our study, one high-ranking law enforcement official stated that, "L.A. is not a brothel town." A few brothels existed, of course, and one citywide vice detective told us that they had just followed a tour bus from the hotels in "Japantown" to a brothel in Hollywood. At the time of our first interviews, police had few leads and no complaints, good indicators that the brothel business was not booming inside the city proper. Prostitution experts from LAPD's Organized Vice and Crime say this generalization still holds true today. Vice detectives with the LA County Sheriff's Department, however, tell a different story. In the Asian community, brothels, passing themselves off as private (i.e., unlicensed) "massage parlors" and "clubs," are run out of homes and apartments, mostly by Koreans, Taiwanese, and Vietnamese. These establishments obtain clients mostly through word-of-mouth and by advertising in the Asian-language papers. Reports in the *Los Angeles Times* suggest that there are Asian prostitution rings that use Latina prostitutes, too (Liu, 1999).

"B & D" (bondage and discipline) and "S & M" (sadomasochism) houses offer services that straddle the line between prostitution and legal consensual behavior. One such place, for example, advertises on its Web site as the only establishment in the City of LA with a sexual encounter license, which means that a "fully nude staff member," almost always a White woman, can provide "full BD/SM contact." A 30-minute "submission and dominance" session with a female "mistress" costs $100. According to the City Attorney's Office, because genital stimulation is not necessarily involved, such activities are not considered prostitution under the California State Penal Code. Several informants told us that more conventional sexual services can be negotiated both on and off the premises in some of these houses, but they are difficult for law enforcement to police. Given their distaste for that type of undercover work, most detectives admit that B&D houses are a probable venue for prostitution that is largely ignored.

Taxi-Dance Halls. Taxi-dance halls have long thrived in LA, where in 2004 there were 11 establishments that advertised "hostess dancing" within a mile of the downtown Convention Center. In contemporary LA it costs 45 cents a minute (i.e., $27/hour) to have female company, and there is no shortage of men willing to pay the 10-minute minimum; some have been steady customers for over a decade. Officially "dance hostesses," but more aptly called taxi-dancers, the girls asked to dance must pull out time cards and punch the clock.

In the late 1970s, prostitution was more overt because customers could "check out" a girl and leave the premises with her; today, rules prohibit a dancer from leaving the premises with a customer until the dancehall closes. Vice squads patrol undercover because they receive complaints from ex-employees about lewd conduct taking place in dimly lit "TV rooms." The vice squad is often present in the parking lot at closing time to be sure there are no sexual transactions in the cars; however, it is not a crime for the dancers to get a ride home or accept a date with their last customer. An administrative vice detective who patrolled the clubs was quoted as saying that he couldn't think of a single case where a club's management was prosecuted for prostitution, yet it isn't discouraged because it's good for business (Booe, 1990).

A few dancers spoke openly with a young filmmaker about the money they earned meeting clients at hotels after hours where they got $200-$250 for intercourse, the same as the rate at the time in escort services (Haddad, 1991). A female sociologist, employed as a taxi-dancer in Oakland and LA for her participant-observation study, confirmed, "Some California taxi-dancers do engage in prostitution . . . [as] the opportunity to exchange sexual favors for cash definitely exists" (Meckel, 1988, p. 143).

Eight of the taxi-dance halls, like the cantinas, are places for Central American immigrants, both customers and dancers. Two of the downtown hostess dancehalls draw a mixed crowd of White, African-American, Latino, and Asian men, and have mostly White dancers. The one upscale dance club that caters exclusively to Asian businessmen and tourists features a "mama-san" who greets the men, typically seated in groups, and then goes behind a screen and selects one or more "hostesses," mostly blond Americans who say they are aspiring actresses and models, to bring to their table. One who agreed to be interviewed said that no one asks a woman to give sexual favors, but if she doesn't, the "mama-san" will pass her over when selecting someone for a "big spender." But another dancer informant said that during a job interview the "mama-san" asked her, "How far are you willing to go to please your customers?" When she replied, "just dance," she was told to "come back when you are more flexible."

DISCUSSION

Data collected from a wide range of sources show a high degree of racial/ethnic segmentation in LA County's prostitution market, both by mode of soliciting clients and by type of locale. The Asian nightclubs and cantinas for Latino immigrants are currently the main venues of locale-based prostitution. Asian women dominate the massage parlor and brothel industries, and Latina immigrants exclusively work the cantinas. Latina women serve Latino men in the hostess dance clubs, while White women serve a mixed clientele. White women dominate in hotels and in clubs featuring nudity, but those locales, although traditionally associated with off-street prostitution, are not important venues for prostitution in LA. African American women dominate the street, as they do in most U.S. cities with diverse populations.

Our results provide examples of entrepreneurial niches in which ethnic sex workers serve a co-ethnic clientele, as in cantinas. The cantinas of contemporary LA offer an environment that is culturally familiar to Spanish-speaking men from Mexico and Central America, and bar girls are an integral part of that environment. Although they serve a multinational immigrant clientele, cantinas are so specific to the immigrant culture that they do not serve the broader Latino community that includes the American born.

We also find examples of ethnic entrepreneurs who market women's sexual services to a broader clientele. Massage parlors are a prime example; the owners in LA have nearly all been Korean. Organized prostitution has long been marketed in Korea to foreign visitors, including U.S. military personnel beginning in the 1960s and Japanese sex tourists beginning in the 1970s (Lie, 1995). The thriving Korean sex tour industry undoubtedly produced entrepreneurs who were able to transfer marketing practices developed in Korea to the US. Korean women were exported in the 1970s to work in Korean bars in the US that served native-born clients as well as Korean expatriates and traveling businessmen (Lie, 1995).

Our data reaffirm that the vice industry provides work for ethnic immigrant groups and reinforce Light's observation that there is cultural specialization in the marketing of prostitution (Light, 1977). LA's newcomers are part of an industry operated by ethnic entrepreneurs who have created cultural replicas of homeland venues for prostitution or, in the case of taxi-dance halls, resurrected an American immigrant institution. The influx of immigrants, augmented by foreign business travelers, produces a sustained demand, as well as a steady supply of women poised to take the place of those who leave. The relatively powerless Asian and Latina immigrant women who work in the hostess clubs and cantinas appear to be blatantly exploited as sex chattel by middle-class Asian business people and upwardly mobile cantina owners.

Some portion of immigrant sex workers may be there of their own free will, motivated by personal profit, but there is no question that a larger portion have been kept there by deception, intimidation, and/or economic coercion. By contrast, the native-born White sex workers, selling services via ad/referral or hotel and strip clubs, and African American sex workers, dominating street solicitation, both reflect contemporary American gender roles and largely work as independent providers. Male pimps play only a small role in prostitution in LA today.

Global awareness of the problem of international sex trafficking has increased in recent years. Most attention has been focused on the sex tourist trade of Southeast Asia and on the streets and brothels of Western Europe, but the U.S. has also seen a rise in sex trafficking from Asia and Latin America. Congress passed the Trafficking Victims Protection Act in 2000 to help combat this crime. As of mid-2004, there is not one shelter for trafficked persons in the U.S. As home to a larger proportion of Asian and Latino immigrants than any other American city, LA is a focal point for anti-trafficking efforts, and the type of research that we have developed can inform those efforts.

Since the early 1990s, research on prostitution has focused largely on HIV (Farley & Kelly, 2000), with other issues that should be of serious concern from a public health perspective receding into the background. The literature provides evidence that most female prostitutes are a highly vulnerable population at risk of many adverse outcomes in addition to HIV/AIDS. For example, 82% of 130 female street prostitutes interviewed in San Francisco reported having been physically assaulted since entering prostitution, and 68% reported having been raped, often repeatedly (Farley & Barkan, 1998). Not surprisingly, 68% of these same women met criteria for a diagnosis of post-traumatic stress disorder. Other studies confirm that a majority of street prostitutes in U.S. cities experience violence (e.g., El-Bassel et al., 2001; Surratt & Inciardi, 2004). Potterat et al. (2004) examined mortality in a cohort of female prostitutes in Colorado Springs and found that the chance of being murdered was about 1% per year during these women's prostitute careers, making active prostitutes almost 18 times more likely to be murdered than women of similar age and race. Less is known about the risk of violence for women working in off-street venues, but it is clearly a major risk for some (Nemoto et al., 2003).

This type of research can contribute to STI and HIV prevention by revealing potential opportunities for intervention as well as challenges that must be met to intervene successfully. Because off-street prostitution is deeply embedded in racial and ethnic immigrant subcultures, it is critical to design targeted, culturally appropriate interventions (Logan, Cole, & Leukefeld, 2002), informed by an understanding of cultural norms regarding sexuality, gender dynamics, and differential access to socioeconomic power (Laumann & Gagnon, 1995). Interventions may often be successfully targeted at the work environment rather than the sex worker. In a study of female bar workers in the Philippines, Morisky et al. (2002) found that workers were 2.6 times more likely to use condoms consistently if they worked in a bar having a condom use policy as opposed to one that had no such policy in place.

The segment of the off-street prostitution market in which clients meet sex workers in known locations is hidden by fronts of legitimacy that allow participants to deny illegal activities. In a huge, multicultural metropolis like LA County, conventional fieldwork on a large scale would be prohibitively expensive. However, this study reaffirms what Winick and Kinsie (1971) had already demonstrated, that many useful sources of information are available to be tapped. Even though segments of the market operate in different ways, most come under the scrutiny of government agencies, and agency officials were uniformly cooperative in sharing with us what they knew and how they knew it. Systematically examining data from other sources, most notably the regional Yellow Page directories and the sex tabloids, was a valuable supplement to our understanding. The work of others (e.g., Nemoto et al., 2003) shows that researchers who share the racial/ethnic background of a venue's manager and employees can establish rapport and gain access to women for in-depth interviews and surveys. That approach could begin to fill the vacuum in our knowledge of locations like cantinas and Asian hostess bars that are absent from the literature. Finally, our research shows that venues such as strip clubs, that received research attention in the 1970s but have been little studied since, have evolved into a variety of differing forms of adult entertainment that deserve separate attention.

Our study falls short of being comprehensive in either its use of sources or its coverage of market segments. Most notably, the Web became available both as a source of information on prostitution and as a means for its marketing during the course of this study, after our most intensive data collection period had ended. Our limited use of the Web to obtain updates and supplemental information did not begin to tap its potential. The Web provides not only data but also sorting tools that future researchers can use to systematically exploit this invaluable resource and greatly expand our understanding of the advertising stratum. It is possible that research on Web-based marketing of prostitution will reveal other examples of segmentation by race and ethnicity. For example, we were not able to gather data to assess whether ownership of Web-advertised escort services in LA is concentrated in the hands of Russian immigrants, as suggested by law enforcement informants and advertising content.

One final caveat is worth emphasizing. We have focused on market segmentation by race and ethnicity in part because that topic has not previously been addressed in the literature, and it is important. However, the larger point is even more important: prostitution is organized in various ways in different venues, and the specifics of this organization and the setting matter, whether we are trying to understand the behavior of parties who exchange sex for money or design interventions to reduce risk. This may require examination of the roles of multiple parties in the setting. For example, Forsyth and Deshtels (1997), studying strip clubs in Louisiana, Texas, and Virginia, found that managers, bartenders, and waitresses all had an important role in influencing what happened between dancers and customers. Race and ethnicity often play an important part, but only a part, of the cultural and organizational context that should be addressed in prostitution research.

REFERENCES

Albert, A. E., Warner, D. L., & Hatcher, R. A. (1998). Facilitating condom use with clients during commercial sex in Nevada's legal brothels. *American Journal of Public Health*, 88, 643-646.

Allison, A. (1994). *Nightwork: Sexuality, pleasure, and corporate masculinity in a Tokyo hostess club*. Chicago: University of Chicago Press.

Bellis, D. J. (1990). Fear of AIDS and risk reduction among heroin-addicted female street prostitutes: Personal interviews with 72 Southern California subjects. *Journal of Alcohol and Drug Education*, 35(3), 26-37.

Booe, M. (1990, July 15) Taxi dancers. *Los Angeles Times Magazine*, pp. 12-18.

Braun, S. (1989, February 16). For Asians, a ritual sip of home. *Los Angeles Times,* pp. A-1, A3, A25.

Deren, S., Sanchez J., Shedlin, M., Davis, W. R., Beardsley, M., Des Jarlais, D., et al. (1996). HIV risk behaviors among Dominican brothel and street prostitutes in New York City. *AIDS Education and Prevention,* 8, 444-456.

El-Bassel, N., Witte, S. S., Wada, T., Gilbert, L., & Wallace, J. (2001). Correlates of partner violence among female street-based sex workers: Substance abuse, history of childhood abuse, and HIV risks. *AIDS Patient Care and STDs,* 15, 41-51.

Farley, M., & Barkan, H. (1998). Prostitution, violence, and posttraumatic stress disorder. *Women & Health,* 27(3), 37-49.

Farley, M., & Kelly, V. (2000). Prostitution: A critical review of the medical and social sciences literature. *Women & Criminal Justice,* 11(4), 29-64.

Fischer, M. J. & Massey, D. S. (2000). Residential segregation and ethnic enterprise in U.S. metropolitan areas. *Social Problems,* 7(3), 408-424.

Forsyth, C. J., & Deshtels, T. H. (1997). The occupational milieu of the nude dancer. *Deviant Behavior,* 18, 125-142.

Freund, M., Leonard, T. L., & Lee, N. (1989). Sexual behavior of resident street prostitutes with their clients in Camden, New Jersey. *Journal of Sex Research,* 26, 460-478.

Garrison, J. (2003a, September 17). New curbs on strip clubs OKd. *Los Angeles Times,* pp. B1, B10.

Garrison, J. (2003b, November 22). Council repeals its ban on lap dances. *Los Angeles Times,* B1, B16.

Haddad, P. (Director). (1991). *Taxidancer.* [Documentary film]. University of Southern California graduate project.

Hong, L. K., & Duff, R. W. (1997). The center and the peripheral: Functions and locations of dance clubs in Los Angeles. *Journal of Contemporary Ethnography,* 26, 182-201.

Jackson, L., Highcrest, A., & Coates, R.A. (1992). Varied potential risks of HIV infection among prostitutes. *Social Science Medicine,* 35(3), 281-286.

Jones, D. L., Irwin, K. L., Inciardi, J., Bowser, B., Schilling, R., Word, C., et al. (1998). The high-risk sexual practices of crack-smoking sex workers recruited from the streets of three American cities. *Sexually Transmitted Diseases,* 25, 187-193.

Kanouse, D. E., Berry, S. H., Duan, N., Lever, J., Carson, S., Perlman J. F., et al. (1999). Drawing a probability sample of female street prostitutes in Los Angeles County. *Journal of Sex Research,* 36, 45-51.

Kuhns, J. B., Heide, K. M., & Silverman, I. (1992). Substance use/misuse among female prostitutes and female arrestees. *International Journal of the Addictions,* 27, 1283-1292.

Lait, M., & Hubler, S. (1999, June 12). Investigation of prostitution ring attracts IRS interest. *Los Angeles Times,* pp. B1, B5.

Laumann, E., & Gagnon, J. (1995). A sociological perspective on sexual action. In R. Parker and J. Gagnon (Eds.), Conceiving sexuality: Approaches to sex research in a postmodern world (pp. 183-213). New York: Routledge.

Lever, J., & Kanouse, D. E. (1998). Using qualitative methods to study the hidden world of offstreet prostitution in Los Angeles County. In J. E. Elias, V. L.

Bullough, V. Elias, & G. Brewer (Eds.), *Prostitution: On whores, hustlers and johns* (pp. 396-406). New York: Prometheus.

Lie, J. (1995). The transformation of sexual work in 20th-century Korea. *Gender and Society,* 9, 310-327.

Light, I. (1977). The ethnic vice industry, 1880-1944. *American Sociological Review,* 42, 464-479.

Liu, C. (1999, July 1). Prostitutes smuggled into U.S., court told. *Los Angeles Times,* pp. B3, B5.

Logan, T. K., Cole, J., & Leukefeld, C. (2002). Women, sex, and HIV: Social and contextual factors, meta analysis of published interventions, and implications for practice and research. *Psychological Bulletin,*128(6), 851-886.

Los Angeles Almanac (2004). Given Place Publishing Company. Retrieved August 24, 2004 from *http://www.losangelesalmanac.com/topics/Population/index.htm#Ethnic%*

Meckel, M.V. (1988). Continuity and change within a social institution: The role of the taxi-dancer. Unpublished Ph.D. Dissertation, University of Nebraska.

Morin, M. (2002, May 3). Kinky therapy for your back. *Los Angeles Times,* pp. A1, A18.

Morisky, D. E., Peña, M., Tiglao, T. V., & Liu, K. Y. (2002). The impact of the work environment on condom use among female bar workers in the Philippines. *Health Education & Behavior,* 29, 461-472.

Nemoto, T., Operario, D., Takenaka, M., Iwamoto, M., & Le, M. N. (2003). HIV risk among Asian women working at massage parlors in San Francisco. *AIDS Education and Prevention,* 15, 245-256.

Paone, D., Cooper, H., Alperen, J., Shi, Q., & Des Jarlais, D. C. (1999). HIV risk behaviors of current sex workers attending syringe exchange: The experiences of women in five U.S. cities. *AIDS Care,* 11, 269-280.

Potterat, J. J., Brewer, D. D., Muth, S. Q., Rothenberg, R. B., Woodhouse, D. E., Muth, J. B., et al. (2004). Mortality in a long-term open cohort of prostitute women. *American Journal of Epidemiology,* 159, 778-785.

Romero-Daza, N., Weeks, M., & Singer, M. (2003). "Nobody gives a damn if I live or die": Violence, drugs, and street level prostitution in inner-city Hartford, Connecticut. *Medical Anthropology,* 22, 233-259.

Rosenblum, L., Darrow, W., Witte, J., Cohen, J., French, J., Gill, P.S., et al. (1992). Sexual practices in the transmission of Hepatitis B virus and prevalence of Hepatitis Delta virus infection in female prostitutes in the United States. *Journal of the American Medical Association,* 267(18), 2477-2481.

Seidlin, M, Krasinski, K., Bebenroth, D., Itri, V., Paolino, A.M., & Valentine, F. (1988). Prevalence of HIV infection in New York call girls. *Journal of Acquired Immune Deficiency Syndromes,* 1, 150-154.

Surratt, H. L., & Inciardi, J. A. (2004). HIV risk, seropositivity and predictors of infection among homeless and non-homeless women sex workers in Miami, Florida, USA. *AIDS Care,* 16, 594-604.

Thompson, E. E., & Harred, J. L. (1992). Topless dancers: Managing stigma in a deviant occupation. *Deviant Behavior,* 13, 291-311.

Truong, T. (1990). *Sex, money, and morality: Prostitution and tourism in Southeast Asia.* London and New Jersey: Zed Books Ltd.

Williamson, C., & Folaron, G. (2001). Violence, risk, and survival strategies of street prostitution. *Western Journal of Nursing Research, 23,* 463-475.

Winick, C., & Kinsie, P. M. (1971). *The lively commerce: Prostitution in the United States.* Chicago: Quadrangle Books.

Witte, S. S., Wada, T., El-Bassel, N., Gilbert, L., & Wallace, J. (2000). Predictors of female condom use among women exchanging street sex in New York City. *Sexually Transmitted Diseases, 27,* 93-100.

Childhood Sexual Abuse as a Risk Factor for Subsequent Involvement in Sex Work: A Review of Empirical Findings

Evelyn Abramovich, MS

SUMMARY. The following paper is a review of research studies examining the relationship between childhood sexual abuse (CSA) and subsequent involvement in sex work. The vast majority of research studies in this area are conducted on primarily female street-based prostitutes; however, there has been a recent emergence of studies focused on male, predominantly gay/bisexual, participants. Also, more studies have begun to include mixed gender samples and non-sex worker comparison groups. Highlights of the paper include a critique of studies reporting a prevalence of CSA, the intervening effects of family environment, runaway behavior, and abuse characteristics, and a brief overview of research on other sex worker populations. Limitations as well as contributions of current studies are underscored and directions for future research are indicated. *[Article copies available for a fee from The Haworth Document Delivery Service: 1-800-HAWORTH. E-mail address: <docdelivery@haworthpress.com> Website: <http://www.HaworthPress.com> © 2005 by The Haworth Press, Inc. All rights reserved.]*

Evelyn Abramovich is affiliated with the Center for Psychological Studies, Nova Southeastern University; the Department of Psychiatry and Health Behavior, Medical College of Georgia, 3488 Castlehill Court, Tucker, GA 30084; and the Augusta Department of Veteran Affairs (E-mail: Eabram99@aol.com).

[Haworth co-indexing entry note]: "Childhood Sexual Abuse as a Risk Factor for Subsequent Involvement in Sex Work: A Review of Empirical Findings." Abramovich, Evelyn. Co-published simultaneously in *Journal of Psychology & Human Sexuality* (The Haworth Press, Inc.) Vol. 17, No. 1/2, 2005, pp. 131-146; and: *Contemporary Research on Sex Work* (ed: Jeffrey T. Parsons) The Haworth Press, Inc., 2005, pp. 131-146. Single or multiple copies of this article are available for a fee from The Haworth Document Delivery Service [1-800-HAWORTH, 9:00 a.m. - 5:00 p.m. (EST). E-mail address: docdelivery@haworthpress.com].

KEYWORDS. Childhood sexual abuse, sex work, exotic dancer, escort, adult film actor

Over the last two decades, an increased interest has developed surrounding the relationship between childhood sexual abuse (CSA) and subsequent involvement in prostitution. Studies on both male and female prostitutes have reported high prevalence rates (i.e., more than half the sample) of CSA among their samples of adults and adolescents. Moreover, a large body of child literature (e.g., Einbender & Friedrich, 1989; Gale, Thompson, Moran, & Sack, 1988; Mian, Marton, & LeBaron, 1996; Young, Bergandi, & Titus, 1994) has consistently and unequivocally shown evidence of a sexualized behavioral pattern following sexual abuse that in some cases persists, if not worsens, over time (Tebbutt, Swanston, Oates, & O'Toole, 1997). However, the research also describes how abuse characteristics (Beitchman et al., 1991; Mian et al., 1996; Ruggerio et al., 2000; Tyler, 2002) and family environment variables (Gray et al., 1999) can be moderating variables by either exacerbating symptoms or curbing them. Studies on adult survivors of CSA indicate that sexual problems, including sexual aversion, sexual dysfunction, sexual compulsivity, sexual preoccupation, and risky sexual behavior (Beitchman et al., 1992; Cahill et al., 1991; Davis & Petretic-Jackson, 2000; Noll, Trickett, & Putnam, 2003) are a common complaint. The conclusion that is often drawn when considering these different bodies of literature collectively is that early sexualization as a result of CSA is reinforced and perpetuated over the lifespan and expressed in adulthood in the form of promiscuity, sexual addiction, and/or prostitution (Kendall-Tackett, Williams, & Finkelhor, 1993).

The objective of the following paper is to examine and review the existing literature on CSA and sex work. In general, researchers tend to disagree as to whether sexual abuse alone versus a more global combination of risk factors (e.g., family characteristics, socioeconomic status, runaway behavior, education level, etc.) is predictive of involvement in prostitution. The limited research in this area has focused primarily on street-based female prostitutes. The few studies that have examined CSA and subsequent prostitution among males have done so within the larger context of risks for HIV or sexually transmitted infections (STIs) and substance use. Studies with mixed gender samples tend to have a higher proportion of females to males.

The majority of articles reviewed in this paper are studies on adult and adolescent female and male prostitutes. However, a comprehensive

literature search utilizing a database of peer-reviewed psychology journals was conducted to find any studies related to CSA and sex work in
general, including prostitution, exotic dancing, and acting in adult pornographic films. Only empirical studies were included in the review. No
articles relevant to the topic were found before the year 1980. Although
some studies reviewed are quite dated and should be interpreted with
caution, it is important to include older studies to examine changes in
trends across the research.

Due to the various phrases and labels used to identify or describe sex
work occupations, several different combinations of keywords were
used to conduct the literature search. As mentioned above, the search resulted mostly in studies that utilized female prostitutes as their participants. For example, entering the keywords "childhood sexual abuse"
and "prostitution" yielded 20 results. Of these results, 10 articles were
deemed to be appropriate and directly related to the topic. Out of these,
only one of the studies utilized male prostitutes as participants. To obtain information on CSA studies that had been conducted with male sex
workers, the author consulted with other researchers who specialized in
this area. Other keywords that were searched in combination with
"childhood sexual abuse" (e.g., "exotic dancers," "strippers," "male
prostitutes," "adult film actors," "escorts") yielded no results. Entering
the keywords "strippers" and "escorts" did not result in any new articles, but the keyword "male prostitutes" resulted in 48 articles, 2 of
which dealt with CSA and prostitution directly. Entering the keywords
"gay/bisexual" and "prostitution" together resulted in four articles with
one directly related to CSA and sex work among males. The keywords
"exotic dancers" yielded a total of 16 articles, two of which discussed a
history of CSA among female dancers. Although some studies are
likely to have been missed, networking with other researchers indicated
that most of the studies conducted in this area have been included in this
paper.

CHILDHOOD SEXUAL ABUSE AND PROSTITUTION

Female Samples

Much of the research on CSA and sex work has been conducted with
primarily street-based adult and adolescent female prostitutes. Some of
these studies (Bagley & Young, 1987; Silbert & Pines, 1983) have reported a prevalence of CSA that is often two to three times higher than

estimated rates in the general population, which range between 20% and 40% for females depending on the study (Bolen & Scannapieco, 1999; Vogeltanz et al., 1999). Furthermore, many studies (Foti, 1995; Potter et al., 1999; Simmons, 2000; Widom & Kuhns, 1996) that have incorporated a comparison group have found that CSA significantly distinguished prostitutes from their non-prostitute counterparts. Conversely, some researchers (Nadon, Koverola, & Schludermann, 1998; Potterat, Phillips, Rothernberg, & Darrow, 1985) have found that CSA is not prevalent in their samples of prostitutes.

Bagley and Young (1987) conducted a study of 45 female ex-prostitutes and 36 non-prostitute controls from a community sample. In comparison to 28% of the control group, 73% of the ex-prostitutes reported being sexually victimized as children. Furthermore, more than half of the ex-prostitutes indicated that the sexual abuse heavily influenced their decision to enter into prostitution. In terms of their sexual history prior to entering into prostitution, the ex-prostitutes engaged in consensual sexual activity at a young age (46.7% began having intercourse between the ages of 14 and 15), nearly one-third had 20 or more sexual partners, and more than half had begun prostituting before the age of 16. Although the prevalence of CSA was a distinguishing factor, ex-prostitutes differed from control participants along other dimensions as well. The ex-prostitute group was also comprised of more ethnic minorities, was less educated, grew up in larger families, and was more likely to come from inner cities.

Similarly, Silbert and Pines (1983) reported a 60% prevalence rate of CSA among their sample of 200 current and former female adult and adolescent street prostitutes. Moreover, 70% of the respondents reported that the sexual victimization influenced their decision to enter into prostitution. However, the authors of this study and the Bagley and Young (1987) study did not elaborate on how the abuse specifically influenced this decision.

Potter, Martin, and Romans (1999) compared 29 female sex workers to 680 non sex worker controls on demographics and the prevalence of CSA. The control group was chosen from an ongoing study on CSA among a community sample of women. Findings indicate that the sex worker group was significantly more likely than the control group to have experienced penetrative sexual abuse in childhood. The sex workers also differed from controls in that they had completed less education, came from lower SES backgrounds, were more likely to have left home at an early age, and were more likely to have been pregnant before their 19th birthday.

In another study, Foti (1995) examined the link between CSA and prostitution among a sample of 1,240 female detainees in a jail setting. Results indicated that the detainees who had been sexually victimized in childhood engaged in prostitution more than twice as often as nonabused detainees did. A similar study conducted by Simmons (2000) on 122 females who were either living in halfway houses or were incarcerated also examined the relationship between CSA and involvement in prostitution. Findings from the study indicated that women who had been involved in prostitution were significantly more likely to have been sexually abused in childhood than women who had never engaged in prostitution.

As mentioned, a couple of studies resulted in contrasting findings to the above-described studies. For example, Nadon et al. (1998) compared adolescent prostitutes to non-prostitute youth across several different variables, including the prevalence of CSA. The relevance and contribution of this study in particular is its inclusion of a control group that is demographically similar to the target group. The total sample was comprised of 45 female prostitutes and 37 female control participants who were recruited from the same geographic locations. Results indicated no significant differences in the prevalence of CSA between the two groups.

Similarly, a study conducted by Potterat and colleagues (1985) compared a sample of 14 female prostitutes to 15 female controls on various characteristics and life experiences. All had been previously infected or were presently infected with gonorrhea. The objective of the study was to examine how the groups differed and how these differences would impact the way in which prostitutes were approached in the future about preventing the spread of STIs. Out of the 14 prostitutes, only one had been sexually abused in childhood, and in the control group 2 of the 15 participants reported the same. There were, however, some noteworthy differences in this study in comparison to other prostitution studies. Not only was the sample size much smaller in this study than in others, but almost all of the participants were White (i.e., 13/14 prostitutes and 13/15 controls), whereas most of the samples employed in prostitution studies tend to be more ethnically diverse or predominantly comprised of minorities. Also, the overall finding in this study was that prostitutes and non-prostitutes were more similar than different.

Male Samples

In recent years, more researchers have begun to study the relationship between CSA and sex work among male, primarily gay/bisexual, prostitutes and escorts. Studies (e.g., Bartholow et al., 1994; Doll et al., 1992; Jinich et al., 1998) on gay/bisexual males in general indicate that the prevalence of CSA tends to be equal to that of females in the general population.

In a study conducted by Bartholow et al. (1994), 1,001 self-identified adult gay/bisexual males were studied on associated risks of CSA. Participants were recruited from three different clinics for STIs. Approximately one-third (37%) of the sample endorsed a history of CSA. In comparison to nonabused men, the abused males were twice as likely to exchange sex for money, drugs, or other commodities. Moreover, of the abused participants, men whose parents were suspected of substance abuse were more likely to have engaged in prostitution. Also, unlike many of the studies on female prostitutes, the majority of the sample (73%) was White, and one-third of the men had completed college.

Parsons, Bimbi, and Halkitis (2001) examined sexual compulsivity and sexual risk behaviors in a sample of 50 gay/bisexual male Internet-based escorts. Thirteen out of the 50 (26%) participants endorsed a history of CSA. Aside from the small sample size, the researchers suggest that the small proportion of males who endorsed a history of CSA may be related to the possibility that Internet-based escorts are not as likely to have a history of CSA as street-based sex workers. However, the uniqueness of this study is in its use of another segment of the sex worker population–Internet-based escorts. Again, like the Bartholow et al. (1994) study, most of the sample (70%) was White, and approximately two-thirds (64%) had completed college.

In their study of 2,676 gay/bisexual Black and Hispanic males, Diloria, Hartwell, and Hansen (2002) examined the relationship between CSA and risk-taking behaviors. Not unlike other studies on gay/bisexual males, 25% of the overall sample reported CSA. Further, they found that sexually abused participants were more than twice as likely as nonabused males to exchange sexual activity for money and over one and a half times as likely to exchange sex for shelter or something to eat. They also reported more sexual partners and more frequent unprotected sex. Hispanic men were more likely than Black men to endorse a history of CSA.

Lastly, a study conducted by Earls and David (1989) examined the psychosocial backgrounds of 50 male prostitutes and 50 non-prostitute controls. Differences were found in terms of early sexual experiences and sexual orientation. Significantly more prostitutes (30%) than controls (12%) had experienced sexual contact with a family member, and at a significantly younger age (9.7 years versus 15 years, respectively).

With regard to sexual orientation, 52% of the prostitute group in comparison to 0% of the control group reported a homosexual orientation.

Mixed Gender Samples

Some studies (Barkan & Farley, 1998; Earls & David, 1990; Widom & Kuhns, 1996; Zierler et al., 1991) have included both male and female sex workers in the same sample; however, comparisons were more often conducted with control participants rather than within the target sample. For example, Farley and Barkan (1998) conducted a study to examine the prevalence and history of violence and PTSD among street-based sex workers. Participants were 130 prostitutes in the San Francisco area; seventy-five percent of the total sample was comprised of female participants, 13% were males, and 12% were transgendered. The authors found that 57% of the participants had been sexually victimized in childhood. However, this percentage was not broken down by gender, preventing further comparisons.

Earls and David (1990) conducted a study comparing the family background and early sexual experiences of 100 male and female prostitutes to 100 male and female non-prostitutes. Unlike other prostitution studies, these authors were able to achieve equal sample sizes of both males and females. Thirty percent of male prostitutes and 26% of female prostitutes reported having sexual contact with a family member at average ages of 9.7 and 10.3, respectively. In the control group, however, only 12% of males and 6% of females reported having sexual contact with a family member at average ages of 14.6 and 11.5, respectively.

In a study conducted by Zierler et al. (1991), sexually abused male and female adults were compared to nonabused males and females to examine whether CSA increases the risk for HIV infection. Overall, approximately 50% of females and 20% of males endorsed a history of CSA. Abused participants in general were found to be four times more likely to engage in prostitution than their respective nonabused counterparts. For sexually abused males, all of whom reported having bisexual experiences, the likelihood of involvement in prostitution was 8 times higher than for nonabused males.

Fiorentine, Pilati, and Hillhouse (1999) conducted a drug treatment outcome study to examine the effects of sexual and physical abuse on various behaviors. The sample consisted of 356 male and female outpatients in a drug treatment program. Six months prior to a 24-month drug treatment follow-up, men reporting CSA were more likely to engage in prostitution than other men; however, the same was not true for sexually abused females. The authors hypothesize that the negative outcome for sexually abused males may be greater than for females.

One prospective study that examined gender differences in prostitutes who have been sexually abused was conducted by Widom and Kuhns (1996). Sexually abused and neglected children and control children were recruited and followed into adulthood. In this study, significant findings indicated that CSA predicted prostitution in female participants (10.5%) but not in males (5%). Neglect was also a significant predictor of prostitution for females, but did not achieve significance for males. Furthermore, more females (76) than males (20) comprised the sexually abused group; thus, the overall variance may be attributed to the vast difference in sample sizes. Interestingly, the highest rate of prostitution (12.8%) was found in physically abused females, with the sexually abused (10.5%) and neglected females (9%) following.

FAMILY ENVIRONMENT AND RUNAWAY BEHAVIOR

Although CSA was found to be prevalent in many of the above-described studies, some of these researchers also examined the family context of their participants. Most studies that assessed family environment and social history found that these individuals tended to grow up in broken and disruptive homes. Moreover, a couple of these studies (Nadon et al., 1998; Potterat et al., 1985) found that runaway behavior was a significant factor in predicting involvement in prostitution above and beyond the prevalence of CSA. Some researchers (Nadon et al., 1998; Seng, 1989; Widom & Kuhns, 1996) indicate that juvenile prostitutes in particular have a high rate of running away and report that many of them come from ineffectual family-of-origin environments characterized by family discord, alcohol abuse, physical abuse, neglect (i.e., poor parental supervision and caretaking) and sexual victimization.

For example, Potterat and colleagues (1985) found that only one of the 14 prostitutes they interviewed had actually been sexually abused, but 7 of them admitted to having run away from home up to 6 times; however the non-prostitute comparison group had a similar history of runaway behavior. Also, both the target and comparison groups reported negative relationships with parents and siblings while growing up.

In the Nadon et al. (1998) study running away was significantly more predictive of involvement in prostitution than sexual abuse because, according to the authors, it is often the only means of survival for underage individuals who lack sufficient work experience and education. In this study, adolescent prostitutes were significantly more likely than non-prostitutes to have run away from home and reported doing so for reasons most often related to family disruption. However, no specific family variables, including sexual abuse, were found to be directly linked to involvement in prostitution.

Further, the prospective cohort study by Widom and Kuhns (1996) found that sexually abused children and neglected children were significantly more likely than nonabused and nonneglected controls to engage in prostitution in young adulthood. The finding that neglect was a significant predictor of prostitution irrespective of sexual abuse suggests that a general dysfunctional family environment might be more predictive of prostitution than more overt forms of abuse. This study also examined the mediating effects of running away on childhood trauma and prostitution. They found that the influence of childhood victimization was reduced, albeit remaining a significant predictor, when runaway behavior was controlled. These findings suggest that although sexual abuse is a significant predictor of prostitution, runaway behavior is likely to have intervening effects. On the other hand, in the study of 1,240 female inmates conducted by Foti (1995), sexual abuse was found to be directly related to involvement in prostitution regardless of a history of running away.

In the Bagley and Young (1987) study approximately 75% of the prostitute group, compared with none of the control group, had left their home environments before the age of 16. Their families were characterized by dysfunction, alcohol abuse, and abuse in general. The main reason these participants gave for leaving home was sexual abuse.

In the Earls and David (1990) study the male prostitutes were more likely than their non-prostitute counterparts to come from family environments with more frequent parental violence and substance abuse. Additionally, female prostitutes were more likely to be victims of physical violence than their non-prostitute counterparts. Overall, both male and female prostitutes had a more negative perception of their family-of-origin environments and had left home at an earlier age than the non-prostitute group; however, no uniform combination of family variables or interaction patterns was identified as predictive of prostitution. In fact, the authors add that leaving home at an early age and having to find a means for survival coupled with an early exposure to sexual experiences might be a more comprehensive explanation for involvement in prostitution than either alone.

ABUSE CHARACTERISTICS

In the child literature, abuse characteristics have been found to have a large influence on whether or not a sexualized behavioral pattern will develop following abuse (Beitchman et al., 1991; Mian et al., 1996; Ruggerio et al., 2000; Tyler, 2002). Similarly, a few studies on prostitutes have minimally examined the role of specific abuse characteristics and their ability to predict involvement in prostitution. For example, Silbert and Pines (1983) reported frequencies of abuse variables (i.e., frequency and severity of abuse, relationship to perpetrator, use of force, etc.) in their study of 200 female prostitutes. Of the 60% of participants who reported CSA, 49% had been victimized repeatedly, 90% were close to or knew their perpetrator, 33% were physically forced and emotionally coerced, and 59% experienced vaginal penetration.

In the Bagley and Young (1987) study the ex-prostitutes differed dramatically from the community sample in the nature of the sexual abuse in that they had endured more severe and frequent victimization, as well as for a longer duration. They also were involved in a wider array of sexual acts, including sado-masochism and posing in pornographic films. Approximately 75% of the prostitutes had been vaginally penetrated, compared to 11% of the control participants. Also, more than half of the target sample indicated that the sexual abuse, although generating negative attitudes toward sex, was consequential in their decision to become a prostitute.

Conversely, in the study conducted by Foti (1995), specific abuse characteristics including severity and relationship to perpetrator did not significantly predict involvement in prostitution although being sexually abused in general did. Similarly, Nadon and colleagues (1998) examined the effects of sexual abuse frequency, duration, and use of force on involvement in prostitution in their sample of adolescent prostitutes and nonprostitutes. Findings from this study indicated that abuse variables failed to significantly distinguish the two groups.

OTHER SEX WORKER GROUPS

Other sex worker populations (e.g., exotic dancers/stripteasers, adult film actors, etc.) have not been widely researched, and this gap in the literature is likely due to the difficulty in accessing these individuals. However, one exception is a study conducted by Ross and colleagues (1990) on 20 patients with multiple personality disorder (known more commonly today as dissociative identity disorder–DID), 20 exotic dancers, and 20 prostitutes. The purpose of the study was to compare the frequency of CSA and current dissociative symtomatology (confusion of memory and/or identity) among these groups. Findings from this study showed that exotic dancers and prostitutes were equally as likely as the DID patients to have experienced CSA (13, 11, and 16, respectively). However, patients with DID reported a significantly longer duration of sexual abuse, more perpetrators, and more types of sexual abuse than the other two groups. No information was obtained about the family backgrounds of any of the individuals in the sample. Therefore, it was not possible to examine the influence of family environment versus sexual abuse characteristics on sex work. Findings from this study also indicate that the exotic dancers and prostitutes were experiencing dissociative symptoms as measured by the Dissociative Disorders Interview Schedule (diagnostic tool) and the Dissociative Experiences Scale (screening instrument). Seven exotic dancers and one prostitute met *DSM-III-R* criteria for DID, and seven prostitutes met the diagnostic criteria for psychogenic amnesia. This is the only study to date that has compared data among different types of sex workers in any domain.

DISCUSSION

Although much can be learned about the relationship between CSA and sex work from the studies described in this review, several limitations and methodological flaws should be noted when considering their findings. What these studies collectively suggest is that although sexual abuse is common among female prostitutes, it is not evident that these individuals have chosen prostitution as a result of being sexualized at a young age. Rather, this research seems to suggest that these individuals are attempting to flee from chaotic family circumstances and are utilizing prostitution for financial livelihood.

The principal flaws in the research as a whole is the use of biased, nonrandom samples and the lack of appropriate, or any, comparison groups. Nadon et al. (1998) argue that perhaps some of the studies that found significant differences between prostitutes and non-prostitutes did not use appropriate controls or underestimated the prevalence of CSA among the general population of youth. Also, a remarkable difference among the studies is that they varied greatly in the composition and demographics of their samples. Some studies recruited predominantly minority samples, while others employed mostly White participants. The participants also varied along education, SES, and geography. Consequently, it is difficult to compare findings from one study to another. However, what this variance indicates is that sex workers in general tend to be a very large and diverse group of individuals who represent various ethnic groups, education levels, life experiences, and so on. It should be noted, though, that these studies used samples that were conveniently available because the sex worker population in general is a very difficult group to access, and it is not likely that large, random samples are realistically achievable.

Another methodological limitation of many of these studies is that very little, if any, data were collected on the nature of the sexual abuse and whether or not behavioral consequences (i.e., sexual acting-out) developed following abuse and continued into adolescence and adulthood. Thus, it is not possible to ascertain if any sexualized behavioral pattern emerged in childhood and how this might have influenced sexual development and subsequent involvement in prostitution. Furthermore, simply inquiring about the presence of a sexual abuse history in sex workers is not sufficient support for the hypothesis that sexual abuse leads to prostitution. Future research should be aimed at collecting more data about not only the nature of the abuse reported, but also symptom development following abuse, treatment received, and the existence of any longstanding sexual behavioral pattern throughout life.

Also, the research on sex workers primarily focuses on female street prostitutes, which is only one small, and often severely disadvantaged, segment of individuals working in the sex industry. Consequently, sexual abuse may be only one of many variables related to their entrance into prostitution. Moreover, many studies utilize samples of individuals that are overwhelmingly impoverished ethnic minorities and/or incarcerated, which makes generalizability to all sex workers even more tenuous. What correlational, much less causal, inferences that can be extrapolated from this body of research shed little light on what can be understood about the larger population of sex industry workers (e.g., exotic dancers, adult film actors, escorts, etc.). As mentioned, these biased samples are largely due to the fact that street prostitutes are a more easily accessible population of sex workers (Bagley & Young, 1987).

Another major gap in the literature on sexual abuse and subsequent involvement in sex work is the absence of data collected on other sex worker populations (i.e., exotic dancers, adult film actors, escorts, legalized prostitutes, etc.). Intuitively, these occupations are not necessarily mutually exclusive groups, and therefore, some differences as well as commonalties are likely to exist among them (e.g., safety, work environment, socioeconomic status, income, etc.). Although it is true that prostitutes might share commonalties with other sex worker populations in the nature of their work, they are also very likely to be demographically dissimilar. The link between sexual abuse and sex work, if in fact it exists, can be solidified if similar trends observed in prostitutes' backgrounds are also noted in other sex worker populations. The current literature on other sex worker populations does not encompass issues relating to sexual abuse. Not unlike the research on male prostitutes, studies on female and male exotic dancers–or stripteasers as they are referred to in the literature–surround various topics including the socialization of becoming a stripteaser (Dressel & Petersen, 1982; Lewis, 1998), occupational characteristics (Forsyth & Deshotels, 1997), customer interactions (Boles & Garbin, 1974), and self-identification (Peretti & O'Connor, 1989) to name a few. Furthermore, research on pornographic films focuses primarily on themes of characters and the consumers who view this material. To date, no known empirical research is available on the individuals acting in adult pornographic films. Since street-based prostitutes are currently the only population of sex workers being widely researched, it cannot be confirmed that sexual abuse alone leads to involvement in sex work.

The current research also provides very little information about gender differences in sexual abuse histories of prostitutes. In most of the above-named studies, males and females were compared to a nonabused or non-prostitute control group more so than with each other. Future studies that are able to employ samples of both males and females might find it beneficial to look at gender differences within the same target group (i.e., prostitutes). This gap in the literature is also largely due to the fact that the existence and accessibility of females to males is disproportionate at best. The availability of male participants is nil in comparison to females, and the content of male studies is typically focused around HIV, associated risk-taking behaviors and substance use. Therefore, if male participants are accessible, accurate and generalizable comparisons to females are unlikely to be forthcoming. Further, since the profession is largely dominated by females, it is unlikely that equal numbers of both genders is attainable. What is more, the vast majority of studies on male prostitutes in general tend to focus on social issues not germane to the topic of sexual abuse. Some of these research topics include sexual behavior (Pleak & Meyer-Bahlburg, 1990), sexual orientation (Cates, 1989; Hoffman, 1972), dynamics of the client-prostitute relationship (Caukins & Coombs, 1976; Luckenbill, 1984), and demographic and personality variables (Cates & Markley, 1992).

Despite some of the drawbacks in the current literature on CSA and sex work, recent studies have made an important step forward toward broadening our understanding of this relationship. Two salient contributions that add to the growth of this research are that studies are beginning to employ more diverse samples by including transgendered participants, sex workers other than street prostitutes, and males. If the accessibility to these other groups is increased, it will hopefully set the stage for future studies to expand their search for participants who are more representative of the entire sex worker population.

REFERENCES

Bagley, C., & Young, L. (1987). Juvenile prostitution and child sexual abuse: A controlled study. *Canadian Journal of Community Mental Health, 6*, 5-26.

Bartholow, B. N., Doll, L. S., Joy, D., Douglas, J. M., Jr., Bolan, G., Harrison, J. S., et al., (1994). Emotional, behavioral, and HIV risks associated with sexual abuse among adult homosexual and bisexual men. *Child Abuse & Neglect, 18*, 747-761.

Beitchman, J. H., Zucker, K. J., Hood, J. E., DaCosta, G. A., & Akman, D. (1991). A review of the short-term effects of child sexual abuse. *Child Abuse & Neglect, 15*, 537-556.

Beitchman, J. H., Zucker, K. J., Hood, J. E., DaCosta, G. A., Akman, D., & Cassavia, E. (1992). A review of the long-term effects of child sexual abuse. *Child Abuse & Neglect, 16*, 101-118.

Bolen, R. M., & Scannapieco, M. (1999). Prevalence of child sexual abuse: A corrective metaanalysis. *Social Service Review*, 281-299.

Boles, J., & Garbin, A. P. (1974). The strip club and the stripper-customer patterns of interaction. *Sociology & Social Research, 58*(2), 136-144.

Cahill, C., Llewelyn, S. P., & Pearson, C. (1991). Long-term effects of sexual abuse which occurred in childhood: A review. *British Journal of Clinical Psychology, 30*, 117-130.

Cates, J. A., (1989). Adolescent male prostitute by choice. *Child & Adolescent Social Work Journal, 6*(2), 151-156.

Cates, J. A., & Markley, J. (1992). Demographic, clinical, and personality variables associated with male prostitution by choice. *Adolescence, 27*(107), 695-706.

Caukins, S. E., & Coombs, N. R. (1976). The psychodynamics of male prostitution. *American Journal of Psychotherapy, 30*(3), 441-451.

Davis, J. L., & Petretic-Jackson, P. A. (2000). The impact of child sexual abuse on adult interpersonal functioning: A review and synthesis of the empirical literature. *Aggression and Violent Behavior, 5*, 291-328.

Diloria, C., Hartwell, T., & Hansen, N. (2002). Childhood sexual abuse and risk behaviors among men at high risk for HIV infection. *American Journal of Public Health, 92*, 214-219.

Doll, L.S., Joy, D., Bartholow, B. N., Harrison, J. S., Bolan, G., Douglas, J. M., et al. (1992). Self-reported childhood and adolescent sexual abuse among adult homosexual and bisexual men. *Child Abuse & Neglect, 16,* 855-864.

Dressel, P. L., & Petersen, D. M. (1982). Becoming a male stripper: Recruitment, socialization, and ideological development. *Work & Occupations, 9*(3), 387-406.

Earls, C. M., & David, H. (1989). A psychosocial study of male prostitution. *Archives of Sexual Behavior, 18*(3), 401-419.

Earls, C. M, & David, H. (1990). Early family and sexual experiences of male and female prostitutes. *Canada's Mental Health, 38*(4), 7-11.

Einbender, A. J., & Freidrich, W. N. (1989). Psychological functioning and behavior of sexually abused girls. *Journal of Consulting and Clinical Psychology, 57*(1), 155-157.

Farley, M., & Barkan, H. (1998). Prostitution, violence, and posttraumatic stress disorder. *Women & Health, 27*(3), 37-49.

Fiorentine, R., Pilati, M. L., & Hillhouse, M. P. (1999). Drug treatment outcomes: Investigating the long-term effects of sexual and physical abuse histories. *Journal of Psychoactive Drugs, 31*(4), 363-372.

Forsyth, C. J., & Deshotels, T. H. (1997). The occupational milieu of the nude dancer. *Deviant Behavior, 18*(2), 125-142.

Foti, S. M. (1995). Child sexual abuse as a precursor to prostitution. *Dissertation Abstracts International: Section B: The Sciences & Engineering, 55*(8-B), 3586.

Gale, J., Thompson, R. J., Moran, T., & Sack, W. H. (1988). Sexual abuse in young children: its clinical presentation and characteristic patterns. *Child Abuse & Neglect, 12,* 163-170.

Gray, A., Pithers, W. D., Busconi, A., & Houchens, P. (1999). Developmental and etiological characteristics of children with sexual behavior problems: Treatment implications. *Child Abuse & Neglect, 23*(6), 601-621.

Hoffman, M. (1972). The male prostitute. *Sexual Behavior, 2*(8), 16-21.

Jinich, S., Paul, J. P., Stall, R., Acree, M., Kegeles, S., Hoff, C., & Coates, T. J. (1998). Childhood sexual abuse and HIV risk-taking behavior among gay and bisexual men. *AIDS and Behavior, 2*(1), 41-51.

Kendall-Tackett, K. A., Williams, L. M., & Finkelhor, D. (1993). Impact of sexual abuse on children: A review and synthesis of recent empirical studies. *Psychological Bulletin, 113*(1), 164-180.

Lewis, J. (1998). Learning to strip: The socialization experiences of exotic dancers. *Canadian Journal of Human Sexuality, 7*(1), 51-66.

Luckenbill, D. F. (1984). Dynamics of the deviant sale. *Deviant Behavior, 5*(1-4), 337-353.

Mian, M., Marton, P., & LeBaron, D. (1996). The effects of sexual abuse on 3-to 5-year-old girls. *Child Abuse & Neglect, 20*(8), 731-745.

Nadon, S. M., Koverola, C., & Schludermann, E. H. (1998). Antecedents to prostitution: Childhood victimization. *Journal of Interpersonal Violence, 13*(2), 206-221.

Parsons, J. T., Bimbi, D., & Halkitis, P. N. (2001). Sexual compulsivity among gay/bisexual male escorts who advertise on the Internet. *Sexual Addiction & Compulsivity, 8,* 101-112.

Potter, K., Martin, J., & Romans, S. (1999). Early developmental experiences of female sex workers: A comparative study. *Australian & New Zealand Journal of Psychiatry, 33*(6), 935-940.

Potterat, J. J., Phillips, L., Rothenberg, R. B., & Darrow, W. (1985). On becoming a prostitute: An exploratory case-comparison study. *Journal of Sex Research, 21,* 329-335.

Noll, J. G., Trickett, P. K., & Putnam, F. W. (2003). A prospective investigation of the impact of childhood sexual abuse on the development of sexuality. *Journal of Consulting and Clinical Psychology, 71*(3), 575-586.

Peretti, P., & O'Connor, P. (1989). Effects of incongruence between the perceived self and the ideal self on emotional stability of stripteasers. *Social Behavior &Personality, 17,* 81-92.

Pleak, R. R., & Meyer-Bahlburg, H. F. (1990). Sexual behavior and AIDS knowledge of young male prostitutes in Manhattan. *Journal of Sex Research, 27*(4), 557-587.

Ross, C. A., Anderson, G., Heber, S., & Norton, G. R. (1990). Dissociation and abuse among multiple-personality patients, prostitutes, and exotic dancers. *Hospital and Community Psychology, 41*(3), 328-330.

Ruggerio, K. J., McLeer, S. V., & Dixon, J. F. (2000). Sexual abuse characteristics associated with survivor psychopathology. *Child Abuse & Neglect, 24*(7), 961-964.

Seng, M. J. (1989). Child sexual abuse and adolescent prostitution: A comparative analysis. *Adolescence, 24*(95), 665-675.

Silbert, M. H., & Pines, A. M. (1983). Early sexual exploitation as an influence in prostitution. *Social Work, 28*(4), 285-289.

Simmons, R. V. (2000). Child sexual trauma and female prostitution. *Dissertation Abstracts International: Section B: The Sciences & Engineering, 61*(2-B), 1096.

Tebbutt, J., Swanston, H., Oates, K., & O'Toole, B. (1997). Five years after child sexual abuse: Persisting dysfunction and problems of prediction. *Journal of the American Academy of Child & Adolescent Psychiatry, 36*(3), 330-339.

Tyler, K. A. (2002). Social and emotional outcomes of childhood sexual abuse: A review of recent research. *Aggression and Violent Behavior, 7,* 567-589.

Vogeltanz, N. D., Wilsnack, S. C., Harris, T. R., Wilsnack, R. W., Wonderlich, S. A., & Kristjanson, A. F. (1999). Prevalence and risk factors for childhood sexual abuse in women: National survey findings. *Child Abuse & Neglect, 23*(6), 579-592.

Widom, C. S., & Kuhns, J. B. (1996). Childhood victimization and subsequent risk for promiscuity, prostitution, and teenage pregnancy: A prospective study. *American Journal of Public Health, 86*(11), 1607-1612.

Young, R. E., Bergandi, T. A., & Titus, T. G. (1994). Comparison of the effects of sexual abuse on male and female latency aged children. *Journal of Interpersonal Violence, 9*(3), 291-306.

Zierler, S., Feingold, L., Laufer, D., Velentgas, P., Kantrowitz-Gordon, I., & Mayer, K. (1991). Adult survivors of childhood sexual abuse and subsequent risk of HIV infection. *American Journal of Public Health, 81*(5), 572-575.

Managing Risk and Safety on the Job: The Experiences of Canadian Sex Workers

Jacqueline Lewis, PhD
Eleanor Maticka-Tyndale, PhD
Frances Shaver, PhD
Heather Schramm, MPhil

SUMMARY. This paper reports results from a study of sex work occupations conducted in a large city in Canada that included women, men, and transsexual/transgender (TS/TG) sex workers. Descriptions of work provided by participants (escorts, exotic dancers, masseuses, and street workers) were used to examine how risk and safety were experienced and managed within the Canadian legal context. Three dimensions of the structure of sex work were identified as factors that influenced the man-

---

Jacqueline Lewis and Eleanor Maticka-Tyndale are affiliated with the Department of Sociology and Anthropology, University of Windsor, 401 Sunset Avenue, Ontario, Canada N9B 3P4 (E-mail: lewis3@uwindsor.ca). Frances Shaver is affiliated with Concordia University. Heather Schramm was a doctoral student at the University of Toronto when this study was conducted.

This project was funded by the Social Sciences and Humanities Research Council of Canada (SSHRC) and the National Network on Environments and Women's Health (NNEWH). The authors would like to thank all the sex workers who participated in the project, who gave their time and shared their experiences. They also wish to thank the following individuals and groups who contributed to the various phases of the project: Kara Gillies, Robert Johnson, Mary Taylor, Jacinthe Brosseau, Megan Street, Laura Wellman, Exotic Dancer's Alliance (EDA), Exotic Dancer's Association of Canada (EDAC), Maggie's, Region of Peel Health, and Stella.

[Haworth co-indexing entry note]: "Managing Risk and Safety on the Job: The Experiences of Canadian Sex Workers." Lewis, Jacqueline et al. Co-published simultaneously in *Journal of Psychology & Human Sexuality* (The Haworth Press, Inc.) Vol. 17, No. 1/2, 2005, pp. 147-167; and: *Contemporary Research on Sex Work* (ed: Jeffrey T. Parsons) The Haworth Press, Inc., 2005, pp. 147-167. Single or multiple copies of this article are available for a fee from The Haworth Document Delivery Service [1-800-HAWORTH, 9:00 a.m. - 5:00 p.m. (EST). E-mail address: docdelivery@haworthpress.com].

agement of risk and safety: its location on- or off-street, its organization on an out- or in-call basis, and whether it was conducted independently or for a club, massage parlor or escort agency. Gender and perceptions of stigma and risk interacted with these dimensions in such a way that men, women and TS/TG workers experienced and managed risk and safety differently. *[Article copies available for a fee from The Haworth Document Delivery Service: 1-800-HAWORTH. E-mail address: <docdelivery@haworthpress. com> Website: <http://www.HaworthPress.com> © 2005 by The Haworth Press, Inc. All rights reserved.]*

KEYWORDS. Sex workers, escorts, exotic dancers, risk, safety

While growing research attention has been paid to sex work in recent years, the focus of this work has been quite narrow. Ignored in the research literature is how social, legal, and economic conditions influence the vulnerability of workers (Shaver, 1997); how sex workers conduct their business and maximize both their income and their safety; the work of men and transsexual or transgender (TS/TG) workers (Weinberg, Shaver, & Williams, 1999), and the relatively invisible forms of sex work (e.g., escorts, exotic masseuses, exotic dancers) (Weitzer, 2000). This paper addresses some of the often-ignored areas, in particular how sex workers experience and manage their work, especially in relation to risk and safety on the job.

Knowledge of Canadian criminal law as it applies to sex work is central to understanding the experiences of Canadian sex workers. The exchange of sex for money is not prohibited by the *Criminal Code of Canada* (1985). While sex work *per se* is not illegal, a number of activities associated with it are. These include: being found in or keeping a common bawdy house (s. 210); providing directions or transporting someone to a bawdy house (s. 211); procuring or living on the avails of prostitution (s. 212); communicating in a public place for the purpose of prostitution (s. 213); and purchasing sexual services from someone under 18 years old (s. 212(4)). In addition, the *Criminal* Code prohibits obscenity (s. 163); immoral theatrical performances (s. 167); indecent acts in a public place (s. 173); and public nudity (s. 174).

Canadian criminal statutes have a different impact on the various forms of sex work. For example, the prohibition on public communication (s. 213) most directly affects street prostitution. Provisions related to bawdy houses (s. 210) make in-call work and sexual contact in strip clubs or massage parlors illegal. Those related to obscenity, indecent acts in a public place, theatrical performances, or public nudity (s. 163, s. 167, s. 173 and s. 174) set legal limits on exotic dancing. The procurement statute (s. 212) limits the use of some strategies that could make escort work safer such as "bringing a friend along on a date." These statutes, however, do not necessarily criminalize out-call activities (those activities that involve the worker going to the client).

In addition to the federal statutes, provincial and municipal legislation deals with vehicular traffic, jaywalking, zoning, and licensing of businesses and occupations. Traffic bylaws have a direct impact on street workers. Zoning bylaws are used to regulate the location of massage parlors, strip clubs, and escort agencies. In addition, a growing number of Canadian cities are using licensing bylaws to regulate who may work and the conditions of work for exotic dancers, escorts, and exotic masseuses. The implications of municipal licensing are discussed in detail in Lewis and Maticka-Tyndale (2000) and Maticka-Tyndale and Lewis (1999).

Although sex work per se is not illegal in Canada, sex workers are neither afforded the rights, nor carry the responsibilities, associated with employment in Canada. They rarely pay income tax, collect taxes from clients, or pay into or receive government benefits such as pension, unemployment, maternity, or compensation for workplace injuries (Lewis & Maticka-Tyndale, 2000; Lippel, Valois, & Shaver, 2002). Few have evidence of employment that can be used in applying for loans or verifying their ability to meet rental, automobile, or other payments. Even when working for a regular employer such as a "strip club" or massage parlour they are typically hired as independent contractors or entertainers, even though their relationship with employers rarely meets federal guidelines for independent contractors (Bindman & Doezema 1997; Lewis & Maticka-Tyndale, 2000; Maticka-Tyndale & Lewis, 1999; Maticka-Tyndale, Lewis, Clark, Zubick, & Young, 1999; 2000). As independent contractors, sex workers are not protected by labor codes or occupational health and safety regulations regarding employer responsibility (Lippel, Valois, & Shaver, 2002).

While sex work itself carries a low social status (Hodgson, 1997; Lowman, 1985-1986), jobs within the industry can be arrayed in a hierarchy. Escorts are located at the top, with their work considered safer (Benoit & Millar, 2001; Lowman, 1985-1986), more lucrative, and easier to hide from public view (Highcrest, 1997; O'Connell Davidson, 1995). Street prostitutes, particularly those who work in the "bad areas" of town, or the "low stroll," make the least money and have the lowest status in this hierarchy. The streets are much riskier than other venues in terms of legal intervention, police arrest, health effects, and experiences of violence, especially that perpetrated by clients (Benoit & Millar, 2001; Jackson, Highcrest, & Coates, 1992; Pyett & Warr, 1997; Whittaker & Hart, 1996). Street-work maintains this dangerous status even when controlling for city, sex worker drug use, duration of drug use, or the age they began sex work (Church, Henderson, Barnard, & Hart, 2001).

While escort work carries the highest status, location at the top of the hierarchy does not necessarily enhance the safety of the work environment. The conditions of work depend, to a great extent, on whether escorts work independently or for an agency. Lewis and Maticka-Tyndale (2000) and Benoit and Millar (2001) found that independent sex workers were in the best relative position to determine their working conditions, including cost of labor, net earnings, pace of work, clientele, and the activities performed while working.

Research on other off-street workers demonstrates that management regulations have a significant impact on the work environment. Those who work in peep shows, where a glass barrier separates them from their audience, have more control over the performer-client relationship than do dancers who work without the safety of a physical barrier. The latter group depends on "tips" from customers and are often fully responsibility for enforcing boundaries between legal and illegal touching (Chapkis, 2000; Maticka-Tyndale et al., 2000). In contrast, for peep show workers, who are physically separated from customers by a glass barrier and paid a wage with no possibility of "tips" from customers, management assumes responsibility for disciplining clientele (Chapkis, 2000).

Reactions to stigma and discrimination, which may also vary by work location, vary by gender. Shaver (1996) argues that the terms given women sex workers (e.g., prostitutes, hookers, whores) carry more stigma than those used for men (e.g., hustlers). And, Browne and Minichiello (1996) argue that women sex workers are bothered more by the stigma and labels of "deviance" than their male counterparts. As a consequence, the women have to put more effort into managing their identities (cited in Vanwesenbeeck, 2001, p. 268). These studies highlight the importance of social and emotional factors in the management of sex work. However, it is external social and organizational factors that create risk and safety. Risks, especially those related to violence, are highest on the streets. Working independently can enhance safety, regardless of the sector.

METHODS

Participants and Procedures

This study was conducted as a collaborative partnership between academics and community partners representing several sex worker organizations and an agency that works with sex workers. The focus was on how public policies influence the working lives, conditions of work, and the health, safety and well-being of sex workers in a large Canadian city. Interviews were conducted with 61 sex workers and 17 key informants between 2000 and 2004, and relevant policy documents were reviewed (e.g., the *Criminal Code of Canada*, municipal regulations and bylaws, social service policies, occupational health and safety and labor codes).

Sex workers were selected using theoretical sampling techniques to maximize diversity in relation to characteristics central to the research questions. Theoretical sampling is a systematic process of selecting participants based on the issues to be addressed, the social circumstances related to them, and an initial estimation of which segments of the population are best able to provide information. Who is interviewed is decided as the research progresses based on the research team's assessment of what has been learned and their judgment of how further information might be gathered (Hammersley & Atkinson, 1989).

The criteria used to establish the parameters for sampling were decided in collaboration with the community partners. Given the primary focus on conditions of work and health, safety and well-being, sex workers were sampled to insure there was representation of those who worked in different settings and forms of sex work, under their own direction and under the direction of someone else, and that were men, women and TS/TG. As the research progressed, we specifically sought out sex workers representing combinations of these characteristics that were, as yet, underrepresented in the sample (e.g., male dancers). Sex workers were recruited through: information about the study that was left in locations they frequented; advertisements in magazines and newspapers distributed to sex workers; a radio show with a sex worker audience; the collaborating partner organizations and their affiliates; referrals from those who were interviewed; and "cold calls" to sex worker advertisements.

All interviews were conducted at a location chosen by the interviewee and were tape-recorded. Interviews were conducted either by one of the academic researchers or a research assistant and lasted between 1 and 4 hours. Once transcribed, interview tapes were destroyed or returned to the interviewee. To preserve the confidentiality of the sex workers who were interviewed, no personal identifying information was obtained, all names and references to specific locations were removed from the interview transcript, and consent to participate was obtained orally. Sex workers were paid a small amount for the interview. We also covered associated transportation and childcare costs. Key informants were not paid for their interviews. Parallel procedures were followed with key informants to preserve confidentiality; however, all key informants were informed that material from their interviews would be identified by their position (e.g., police officer, city councillor, health care provider). The research protocol was reviewed and cleared by the University of Windsor Ethics Review Board.

The sex workers interviewed covered a broad range of occupations: exotic dancing, street prostitution, escort, and massage. Of the 61 interviewed, 30 identified as women, 22 as men and 9 as TS/TG. All were over the age of 18 years. Included in the sample were workers who were single as well as those who were in various forms of relationships, those with and without children, workers who restricted their activity to only one sex work occupation and others who had experience in several, workers who were dependent on sex work for their total livelihood, and those who also had other sources of income. Key informants included 2 city councillors, 2 employees of the city licensing office, 2 police officers, 4 representatives of agencies working with sex workers, and 7 representatives of sex worker advocacy organizations.

Measures

The first drafts of the interview guides were based on prior research on sex work (Lewis & Maticka-Tyndale, 1998; Maticka-Tyndale & Lewis, 1999; Shaver, 1996; Shaver & Weinberg, 2002; Weinberg, Shaver & Williams, 1999). These were reviewed and modified by all collaborating partners (academics and representatives of organizations) and were pilot tested during workshops that trained sex workers as research assistants. Research assistants included graduate students and current and former sex workers; all were trained to conduct interviews and graduate students were trained in coding.

Data Analysis

Scolari N6 was used to code interviews and analyze data. At least two research assistants coded interviews. To insure consistency, coders regularly compared notes. Interviews were initially coded based on the themes included in the interview guides. Those used for this paper included: experiences of work; health and safety threats of work; experiences with poor health and safety on the job; how threats to health and safety are dealt with; organizations, institutions, or individuals and practices that either exacerbate or ameliorate threats to health and safety; and what is liked or enjoyed about the job. Text was coded following the interview schedule as well as the themes identified in the literature and new themes that emerged from the interviews. Text within each theme was compared to identify common and unique patterns based on gender, type of work, and location of work. Results reported here were supported by at least 2 interviews to insure they were not merely idiosyncratic of a single individual or setting. Further, accounts from interviews with different types of participants (e.g., sex workers, community representatives, city officials) and analysis of policy documents were triangulated to increase confidence in the conclusions drawn. The themes from the literature and emerging from interviews were used to organize the presentation of results.

RESULTS

Social Location and Organization of Sex Work

Occupational Hierarchy

The status hierarchy described by other researchers (Brannigan, 1998; Lowman 1985-1986) was evident in the way sex workers we interviewed spoke of themselves and others. This was particularly so in interviews with off-street workers at the upper levels of the occupational hierarchy. Exotic dancers, for example, distanced themselves from sex work by referring to themselves as "performers" rather than sex workers. Dancers and escorts frequently qualified references to other sex workers with comments such as "I'm not like them," "I'm not a prostitute." Even among street prostitutes those who worked in the better areas of town or the "high stroll" differentiated themselves from those on the "low stroll."

The differentials in risk associated with placement on the occupational hierarchy were frequently cited by workers as reasons for leaving lower status jobs, such as those on the street.

> I used to work downtown . . . at the corner and stuff but that's really dangerous. I mean, because you don't know who you're getting. (Female, Escort)

> Getting jumped, getting hurt, . . . getting beat up . . . I was getting tired of it [street work]. I started seeing regulars and stopped jumping into cars. . . . You grow up. . . . I have a lot of friends that are dead now. . . . I want to live safely and I don't think it's safe just to jump in a car. . . . I don't want to die that way. (Female, Escort)

Street workers also differentiated risks by the social location of their work. Greater risk was associated with "low stroll" work.

> The universe is telling me I shouldn't be . . . in [the low stroll] cause it's dangerous. I've been mugged there once. I'm lucky that I'm alive. (Female, Street)

Certain types of street work were also seen as more dangerous.

> I've done hundreds of clients in cars and that is the most dangerous way. . . . I feel more safe when I'm at home or at their place. (Male, Street Worker)

Independent, off-street workers spoke of both greater and lesser vulnerability associated with their work. They did not have access to the protection that agencies or employers provided (e.g., receptionist check-in calls, protection provided by drivers and bouncers). However, they were not bound by agency or employer requirements or regulations that could increase their vulnerability. Instead, independent off-street workers had the freedom to develop their own descriptions and parameters for their work and to establish their own ways of dealing with safety and risk. In contrast, when working with an agency or for an employer, they were typically not in control of the type of work they could do.

Income

The income of sex workers in our sample varied; income was generally higher at night, during tourist season, and when the economy was doing well. Police enforcement practices also influenced income. Shifting between or occupying several sex work occupations was a strategy used to deal with slow business, an unfriendly environment, or a need to make up for income lost as a result of time spent away from work. Some escorts, for example, reported moving to massage parlors or the street when "there weren't many calls coming in." Street workers sometimes moved indoors to strip clubs or massage parlors during "winter months" or when there was "too much heat on the streets" due to police crackdowns. Some exotic dancers regularly turned to escort work to make some "extra cash."

This movement between jobs demonstrated the complex relationship between income, safety, worker preference, and occupational hierarchy. While inside jobs that are further up the hierarchy, such as escort work and exotic dancing, were generally considered safer and to produce higher income, not all workers aspired to these jobs. When faced with economic needs, the shift between occupations was most often from jobs further up the hierarchy to those lower down, which also meant moving from safer to more dangerous work. Some inside workers reported turning to the streets "on a slow night, when the bills were due" despite previous victimization experiences and fear for their "personal safety" or a "general preference" to avoid street work and the "risks that go along with it." Similarly, street workers talked about violating their personal rules and "accepting risky tricks" when they had to make up for "lost money."

Limits to Moving Between Jobs

Movement between various jobs and statuses was not equally available to all workers. Women and men worked both on and off the street. Women reported that they engaged in street prostitution, worked in massage parlours, strip clubs, for escort agencies and did independent escort and massage work. Men also had a number of options. They did street work, provided sexual services in bathhouses and bars or clubs, worked as exotic dancers, and did escort and massage work. Since escort agencies and massage parlors had few requests for male (or TS/TG) workers, when men or TS/TG people worked off-street, they typically worked independently.

TS/TG workers had fewer choices than either women or men. While they listed some of the same work options as men, most worked exclusively on the street. The type of work they engaged in and/or the street location of their work changed as their gender changed. Some TS/TG workers spoke about starting out in "boys town," as male street prostitutes. When they began working as TS/TG women, they moved to the "trannie stroll."

Municipalities that license some forms of sex work also restrict who may be licensed and how the job is done. This was the case for exotic dancers in the city we studied. Those with a recent history of prostitution or drug offences were ineligible for a license, making it impossible for some to move from the more visible (and risky) forms of sex work to exotic dancing. Dancers could also lose their license if they were found to be involved in such activities.

Safety

Discrimination

Prior research has described discrimination against sex workers as rooted in the stigmatization of sex work as well as in its position as an illegitimate occupation (Brock, 1998). Stigma was noted by those we interviewed:

> There's such a stigma attached to prostitutes. [In the public eye] There's nothing worse than prostitution! Being a ho! (Female, Street Worker)

Although all sex workers had to contend with the stigma and discrimination that go along with their job, there were differences in the extent and form of discrimination they had to deal with. The stigma of sex work was *"bounded and temporal"* (Pheterson 1990; 1993) for male workers, restricted almost exclusively to the time they were on the job. The men spoke of stigma and discrimination primarily in association with fear of being recognized or gay bashed while working.

> Believe it or not, I am paranoid that people driving around will recognize me . . . cause not too many people know, believe it or not. I have kept it on such a low key that not too many people even realize it. (Male, Escort/Street Worker)

By comparison, women's experiences of stigma expanded beyond their working lives. Former as well as current women sex workers experienced scrutiny, attack, and police harassment both during and after work.

> Basically [one of the hard parts of the job is] the cops and how they treat you, like you're the worst piece of shit on earth and they bug

you. [It is] Like the man has an effect health-wise on my mind. (Female, Street Worker)

The situation for TS/TG workers was worse than that of men or women. Since they fell outside of commonly accepted concepts of gender, they described themselves as "lack[ing] a legitimate" place in society. The majority of the TS/TG workers felt their gender made them "unemployable," with many supported by government disability pensions. For the TS/TG workers we spoke with, sex work was seen as one of the "few" or the "only option" available to make additional income.

TS/TG workers also reported discrimination in accessing housing and shelter. Several in this study did not have permanent housing, compounding their economic problems. They spoke of needing money to get a place to live and needing an address to receive government disability pension. Even their access to shelters was limited. At the time of this study, there was only one women's shelter that had a bed to accommodate male-to-female (MTF) members of the TS/TG population. When there were no beds for TS/TG women in women's shelters, their only options were a men's shelter–where they risked verbal, physical and sexual harassment and assault–or sleeping on the streets.

Harassment and Assault

The sex workers talked about harassment and assault by both the public and police. This was particularly the case for street workers, especially women and TS/TG workers, who reported persistent harassment by the public. Bottles, food and insults were thrown from passing cars.

> Eggs and bottles against buildings and people screaming out of cars and . . . gay bashers and what have you. You know, that can be scary. (TS/TG, Street Worker)

People living in the neighbourhoods where they worked "threatened" them and tried to "chase" them from the area.

In contrast with street workers, most off-street workers were invisible to the public. As a result, they reported less fear of harassment, abuse, or arrest.

> I know a lot of people who do in-calls [clients coming to the worker] and out-calls from ads and they rarely get beaten up and they rarely get arrested. (Female, Escort)

While they were less visible and less fearful, they did report being subject to inquiries and harassment by "hotel staff," "nosy neighbours," and "busy-body taxi drivers." Some also reported police harassment.

> Cruisers would crawl along the curb next to me when I was going home. I got calls that I interpreted as threatening phone calls. When I picked up the phone, I'd hear like sawing noises or chocking noises. (Female, Masseuse)

In addition to harassment, women talked about police expecting sexual services.

> So the long and the short of it is that internal affairs decided it was my word against the cops in terms of the sexual services [they made me provide] and . . . there was no law or policy against the cops taking sexual services from a prostitute if it was part of a legitimate investigation. (Female, Escort)

Because TS/TG workers were primarily on the streets, they were especially fearful of victimization. Several reported feeling targeted for violent attacks because of the way they looked and where they worked, and, like the men, they were fearful of being "gay bashed." In addition to the stigma associated with their work, they had to contend daily with stigma, harassment, and potential violence resulting from reactions to their TS/TG status. One TS/TG person reported being intentionally hit "by a 2 x 4 extended from a window of a [passing] car." Others spoke of being verbally and physically "harassed" by male pedestrians. In addition, it was emphasized that there was always a potential risk of assault by clients.

The independent workers described their ability to set their own hours, their own limits for what they would and would not do, and the location of their work, as particularly important for maintaining safety. Escorts and masseuses who maintained business apartments or houses and others who saw customers in their own homes described these as important for safety. Although they recognized that they risked arrest by working in a fixed location, this was secondary to the safety and empowerment they felt from controlling their work environment.

> I think on a more subtle level, when somebody is coming to visit you in your space the power dynamic is slightly in your favor. The client is in guest mode and from the minute you open the door to

usher them in, you're directing them here, you're directing them there and you're asserting some control over them, although it's . . . very subtle. Where if you are going into a client's home or hotel, you're in their space, which in addition to the practical dangers . . . you're the guest in their home. (Female, Independent Masseuse)

The independent off-street workers who had regular customers and rarely advertised, reported feeling the farthest removed from potential harassment, violence and victimization by clients.

I have known them [my clients] for years . . . and the girls that I know they just kind of say here is someone that you can call . . . the guy is okay. . . . I find it a lot safer than being out on the street. (Female, Escort)

Because they placed few advertisements they also felt it was difficult for police to detect their activities, minimizing their concern for police intrusion into their lives.

Most of the exotic dancers in the study also worked as "independents." In contrast with other independent workers, however, dancers reported they exercised little control over their environment when working in strip clubs. Since clubs were open to the public, dancers could not restrict access of either clients or police. Police frequented clubs for surveillance related to city bylaw and *Criminal Code* enforcement, and in the process scrutinized the work of dancers. Clients of the clubs were described as posing the greatest risk for harassment and assault in the club and in the parking lot.

Sometimes when I'm going to my car in the parking lot customers will be pulling in. And they feel that because we're on the premises they can start treating me as if I'm at work. I don't want to be spoken to in the parking lot. They don't understand that once I leave the door I'm not working. (Female, Dancer)

Bouncers and club staff provided a layer of protection against clients by "watch[ing] their [dancers'] backs." The reliability of this support was limited, however, by owners and managers who "want[ed] to make their customers happy," and clients that "tip[ped] bouncers to look the other way." Both men and women dancers reported many of the same concerns and both generally felt able to manage their customers.

> Sometimes you have to deal with . . . rude customers. . . . Very
> pushy, and grabby, and they try to . . . put their hands in your pants,
> and all that crap, I'm like, don't do that [so] I pull myself away, or
> slap them on their hand. . . . Don't do that, I don't like it. (Male,
> Dancer)

However, the women were more likely to express concern for their
physical safety than the men were, with men reacting to inappropriate
and assaultive behavior by customers more with irritation than fear.

Rights to Protection

One role of police is to provide protection for citizens from assault or
robbery. The sex workers in our study, however, felt they had little access to police protection and that they received differential treatment
compared to other workers when they were victimized. They were re-
luctant to call police when they were "ripped off" or "rolled," or when
their customers "didn't pay" because they believed that their complaints
would not be taken seriously. Some escort agency owners reported that
police "refused to take action" in cases where customers wouldn't pay
the agreed upon "agency fee" or escorts failed to pay the agency for
"agency services." Men who worked on the street reported an absence
of police assistance in time of need, and an absence of police interest in
them compared to their interest in other forms of sex work.

> They [the police] ignore the boys. It's all about busting the big Ma-
> fia-run agencies. Prostitutes don't disappear from agencies. Boys
> disappear off the street. They're considered runaways and that's
> the end of the story.

It was clear that whether or not police officers actually demonstrated a
"you're just a whore" attitude, sex workers believed they would, and
this kept them from seeking assistance.
   In interviews, police spoke of a commitment on the part of police services in this city to improve their relationship with sex workers. In one
police division, a member of the sex crimes unit acted as police liaison
to the sex worker community. This detective described her job as including "outreach, responding to and investigating the victimization of
sex workers, and encouraging and assisting workers in pressing
charges." Although this is an example of an attempt by police to improve sex workers' access to police protection, it appears likely, based

on the responses of sex workers in our study, that more work will be needed before a working relationship between sex workers and police is established.

Managing Safety

Although threats to safety came from clients, the public and police, when workers discussed strategies for managing their own safety, they spoke almost exclusively about maximizing safety by managing their clients and their business. The business transactions engaged in by all of the sex workers we interviewed, regardless of gender, were predominantly the provision of sexual services to men. While women, men, and TS/TG workers alike spoke of threats to safety from the men they serviced, their reasons differed. Women expressed more concerns about physical and sexual assault, and their ability to protect themselves should a client become violent. Men, especially street workers, also expressed concerns about physical assaults, especially from clients they described as "freak[ing] out" after the sexual transaction.

> I think he just . . . got extra mad . . . and decided to take his anger out of himself for being homosexual or bisexual or whatever, on me, on my head. Some guys are like that . . . they are straight as an arrow in their everyday lives, and they just want to totally go down on a guy. . . . And some of them are very angry at themselves because . . . they're attracted to it. (Male, Escort)

The men most often spoke of feeling confident that they could protect themselves if such a situation arose.

> Because of my size, I feel I could defend myself . . . physically. (Male, Escort)

In contrast, women workers were more likely to rely on others (e.g., other workers, drivers for escorts, and bouncers for exotic dancers) to assist in their protection.

Strategies for dealing with risks varied by venue and gender. Street workers relied on strategies such as "working with a friend" that would "watch out" for them and note the license plate number of the cars they got into. Some relied on intuition and being able to assess customers based on appearance.

> I go on instinct. . . . My instinct is what keeps me safe on the street.
> . . . Their car, the way they look, the way they talk to me, the way
> they stop their car. It could be 10 billion things within a split sec-
> ond [that helps me make my decision]. It's like a bunch of signals
> going off in front of me, like "Oh no! Keep walkin'!" (Female,
> Street Worker)

Others avoided isolated locations, and in some cases avoided cars to minimize risk.

> You just need to . . . stay away from bushes and shit like that, you
> know what I mean? Dark spots. Because it would be easy to be
> pulled right in. (Female, Street Worker)

> If I'm in a person's car, I have no way of being able to get any help. It
> doesn't matter how much you scream. Sometimes in this city [even if
> you scream] people don't pay attention. (Female, Street Worker)

Escorts who used the services of an agency relied on agency check-ins, cell phones, and drivers to provide security protection.

> The driver is there for their [the female escort's] protection.
> They're security guards. If the girl's not out of the house in 50
> minutes, he comes knocking. (Male, Escort)

Men preferred to work in bathhouses or hotels because of the public nature of such settings.

> I feel safer in a bathhouse. . . . There's one that a lot of guys go to
> . . . . They turn a blind eye to it [doing business], so it's pretty cool,
> as long as you don't bother anybody. . . . [With] a bathhouse or a
> motel there's a lot of people around and you can yell if you need to.
> (Male, Escort)

The farther removed from the street and public attention the work was, the safer the workers felt, even though this made them more isolated and less visible to the potentially helpful gaze of others. One man, for example, had a preference for meeting customers in a club.

> There's a bar and you can go in and just sit there and have a drink
> and basically all the older people are clients and all the younger

people are people who work. And basically you can go there and work out your things in the bar and then go back to his place or your place and the transaction's done there. There's an atmosphere where you're not on the street, they're not in their car, you're in a bar. . . . It's safer because . . . the environment is not on the street. (Male, Street Worker/Escort)

Exotic dancers preferred working in clubs where they were familiar with the physical space and knew the staff's responses to potential safety threats. Mirrors on walls were used to track clients who were not in direct view and bouncers were depended on to assist with threatening customers. Other than selecting the clubs they worked in with an eye to the conditions of the establishment and its facilities, dancers generally felt they had no control over these workplace conditions.

DISCUSSION

A focal concern in much of the literature and policy related to sex work is the dangerousness of the work. This is seen as a reason to keep people out of sex work. Our focus has been on the positioning of sex work in Canadian society and how this influenced the experience and management of risk and safety on the job. Several factors come into play. The conduct of both on- and off-street and in-call and out-call work was influenced by the strategies of those enforcing federal criminal statutes and municipal bylaws. The visible presence of street workers was most likely to draw the attention of the police and the public. Thus, they found themselves the most stringently regulated and the most likely to be found violating the *Criminal Code* and municipal bylaws. Those who worked off-street were less visible and their infractions less likely to be detected. The one exception was exotic dancing which occurs off-street in a less visible setting, but which was subjected to increased police scrutiny because of licensing restrictions.

The management of risk and safety on the job was also influenced by its location in the occupational hierarchy, but not in a straightforward manner. Location at the top of the hierarchy in off-street occupations included the possibility of an added layer of protection (e.g., drivers, call-back services, supportive staff). Yet, it did not preclude the owners and managers of these businesses from imposing their own set of rules (e.g., requiring workers to provide certain types of services regardless of their preferences or well-being), thus restricting the ability of workers to maintain their own safety. Working independently, whether off- or on-street, provided the freedom and flexibility to set personal boundaries, but lacked the added layer of protection.

Gender influenced risk management and safety strategies, but did so in interaction with location on the hierarchy and one's organizational opportunities as a dependent or independent worker. Men, because of their physical size, felt confident they could deal with risks to their safety. Although TS/TG workers typically shared the male size advantage, they expressed the greatest concerns for their safety and reported frequent experiences of harassment and assault from both the public and the police. Women fell between these two groups. Since they had access to the largest number of sex work occupations, they were able to move between them in order to maximize their safety and their income.

Fear of discrimination, harassment, and assault were common to all genders and forms of sex work. In part this is because sex workers have stepped outside the social norms and rules governing sex, sexuality, and gender. It is also because sex work is not considered a legitimate occupation. As with any form of behavior that is perceived to violate social and/or occupational norms, there is a cost. For this population, the penalty comes in the form of mistreatment, verbal and physical assault, and lack of access to police services and legal redress. We found, however, that the cost varied across the study population. The TS/TG workers, who fell outside both gender and occupational norms, were subjected to the worst treatment and suffered the most discrimination. Regardless of gender, however, those at the low end of the hierarchy suffered more discrimination and worse treatment than those at the upper end, perhaps indicating a link between location on the hierarchy and perceptions of legitimacy on the part of the public.

The limitations of this research stem from the qualitative nature of its design, our sampling technique, and the population of interest. First, since representative sampling techniques were not used, we cannot report on how common or frequent experiences were. Our sampling technique also meant that we were less likely to access certain kinds of workers. While the workers we interviewed spent varying amounts of time doing sex work and had varying degrees of dependence on the income they earned through this work, all identified themselves as working in this industry. Those who only very occasionally do this work and do not identify with the industry were not accessed through our sampling techniques. We also did not access street workers with "pimps." This could either be because, as some studies conclude, there are few sex workers with pimps (Shaver & Weinberg, 2002), or that having a "pimp" precluded workers from being part of the sample (i.e., the "pimp" didn't want them to participate; they were afraid to participate, etc.). Those who work exclusively in phone-sex work, Internet, or pornography are missing from this research as well, in part because they were less relevant to our research aims. Their jobs typically do not involve coming into direct contact with the public and customers. We had no interviews with workers who reported being trafficked against their will or forced to do sex work. This is likely because of language barriers (interviews were conducted only in English or French) or the inability of these workers to voluntarily come forward for interviews.

The increased knowledge and understanding of the sources of risk for Canadian, urban sex workers that we have gained from this research lead us to five recommendations. Three are oriented to changes in law and/or policy; one focuses on better education, particularly with respect to police/community relations, and the last addresses funding issues. First, to reduce security risks it is important to allow sex workers to provide in-call services legally. This requires modifications to be made to the *Criminal Code of Canada*.

The second recommendation has to do with changes to municipal bylaws in cities that license sex work. There is debate about whether such bylaws have a positive or negative impact on sex workers (Lewis & Maticka-Tyndale, 2000). In the city where we did this research only exotic dancers were licensed. Some other Canadian municipalities, however, also license escort work, body rub, modeling, and/or the provision of certain "personal services." We recommend that municipalities review their existing or potential bylaws from the perspective of including provisions that contribute to the ability of licensed sex workers to conduct their work as safely as possible. We also recommend that those with a history of prostitution related offences not be excluded from obtaining licenses.

The third, and similar, recommendation is that provisions for eligibility for access to protections under existing labor codes, workers' compensation acts, and compensation for victims of crime be reviewed. Sex workers should not be excluded from such provisions. When revising these provisions, care must be taken to ensure that they do not undermine risk-management strategies the sex worker community has already adopted (cf., Lippel et al., 2002).

The fourth recommendation is to increase education opportunities with respect to police/community relations and to create more police/community liaison officers. This would involve developing and establishing mandatory training classes designed to educate police on dealing with marginalized populations. Such classes may help the police deal more sensitively and effectively with the sex worker community. Liaison officers could work to facilitate better police/community (sex worker) relations.

Our final recommendation is to make government funding available for development of communication strategies designed to provide sex workers with information about the laws related to their work, their rights as citizens, and ways to maximize their safety and security on the job. This funding should cover expenses associated with designing and carrying out communication strategies through such vehicles as workshops, meetings, appropriate media, and peer leaders and should elicit the cooperation of appropriate local community and sex worker organizations. Given that readings of risk, perceptions of control, and the experiences of stigma and discrimination vary by gender and the social location and organization of sex work, these groups are in the best position to design population-specific strategies.

REFERENCES

Benoit, C. & Millar, A. (2001) *Working conditions, health status, and exiting experiences of sex workers*. British Columbia Canada: PEERS Prostitutes, Education, Empowerment and Resource Society.

Bindman, J. & Doezema, J. (1997). *Redefining prostitution as sex work on the international agenda*. London: Anti Slavery International and Network of Sex Work Projects.

Brannigan, A. (1998, February). Personal communication.

Brock, D. R. (1998). *Making Work, Making Trouble: Prostitution as a Social Problem*. Toronto: University of Toronto Press.

Chapkis, W. (2000). Power and control in the commercial sex trade. In R. Weitzer *Sex for Sale. Prostitution, Pornography, and the Sex Industry* (pp. 181-201). New York: Routledge.

Church, S., Henderson, M., Barnard, M., & Hart, G. (2001, March). Violence by clients towards female prostitutes in different work settings: Questionnaire survey. *British Medical Journal, 322*(7285), 524-525.

Hammersley, M. & Atikinson, P. (1989). *Ethnography: Principles in Practice*. New York: Routledge.

Highcrest, A. (1997). *At Home on the Stroll: My Twenty Years as a Prostitute in Canada*. Toronto: Alfred A. Knopf.

Hodgson, J. F. (1997). *Games pimps play: Pimps, players and wives-in-law: A quantitative analysis of street prostitution*. Toronto: Canadian Scholars' Press.

Jackson, L., Highcrest, A. & Coates, R.A. (1992). Varied potential risks of HIV infection among prostitutes. *Social Science and Medicine* 35(3) August, 281-86.

Lewis, J. & Maticka-Tyndale, E. (1998) *Erotic/exotic dancing: HIV related risk factors*. Report to Health Canada. *www.uwindsor.ca/star.*

Lewis, J. & Maticka-Tyndale, E. (2000). Licensing sex work: Public policy and women's lives. *Canadian Public Policy, 26*(4), 437-449.

Lippel, K, Valois, G. & Shaver, F.M. (2002). *The sex trade environment part II: Access to compensation for workers in the sex industry who are victims of crime.* Final Report submitted to the National Network on Environments and Women's Health (August 10).

Lowman, J. (1985-86, Dec-Jan). Prostitution in Canada. *Resources for Feminist Research, 14*(4), 35-37.

Maticka-Tyndale, E. & Lewis, J. (1999) *Escort services in a border town: Transmission dynamics of sexually transmitted infections within and between communities.* Report prepared for Laboratory Centres for Disease Control, Division of STDs and HIV.

Maticka-Tyndale, E., Lewis, J., Clark, J., Zubick, J. & Young, S. (1999). Social and cultural vulnerability to sexually-transmitted infection: The work of exotic dancers. *Canadian Journal of Public Health,* 90(1), 19-22.

Maticka-Tyndale, E., Lewis, J., Clark, J., Zubick, J. & Young, S. (2000). Exotic dancing and health. *Women & Health, 31*(1), 87-108.

O'Connell Davidson, J. (1995) The anatomy of "free choice" prostitution. *Gender, Work and Organization, 2,* 1-10.

Pheterson, G. (1990). The category "prostitute" in scientific inquiry. *The Journal of Sex Research, 27*(3), 397- 407.

Pheterson, G. (1993). The whore stigma: Female dishonor and male unworthiness. *Social Text,* 37, 39-64.

Pyett, P.M. & Warr, D.J. (1997). Vulnerability on the streets: Female sex workers and HIV risk. *AIDSCare,* 9(5) October, 539-547.

Shaver, F.M. (1996). Prostitution: On the dark side of the service industry. In T. Fleming (Ed.) *Post Critical Criminology* (pp. 42-55). Scarborough, ON: Prentice Hall.

Shaver, F.M. (1997). *Occupational health and safety on the dark side of the service industry: Findings and policy implications.* International Conference on Prostitution. Los Angeles, CA. (March).

Shaver, F.M. & Weinberg, M. (2002). *Outing the stereotypes: A comparison of high track strolls in Montreal, Toronto, and San Francisco.* Paper presented at The Society for the Scientific Study of Sex, Annual Meeting. Montreal, QC.

Vanwesenbeeck, I. (2001). Another decade of social scientific research on sex work: A review of research 1990-2000. *Annual-Review-of-Sex-Research, 12,* 242-289.

Vazquez, A., & Martin. (1996) *Coercion: An important factor restricting access of drug users and sex workers to the health system.* Presented at the XI International Conference on AIDS, Vancouver, BC., [We.D.495]).

Weinberg, M. S., Shaver, F.M. & Williams, C.J. (1999). Gendered sex work in the San Francisco tenderloin. *Archives of Sexual Behavior,* 28(6), 503-521.

Weitzer, R. (2000). Why we need more research on sex work. In R. Weitzer (Ed), *Sex for Sale: Prostitution, Pornography, and the Sex Industry* (pp. 1-13). New York: Routledge.

Whittaker, D. & Graham, H. (1996). Research note: Managing risks–the social organization of indoor sex work. *Sociology of Health and Illness,* 18 (3), 399-414.

Strategies of Stigma Resistance Among Canadian Gay-Identified Sex Workers

Todd G. Morrison, PhD
Bruce W. Whitehead

SUMMARY. The purpose of the current study was to explore how sex workers (specifically, gay-identified Canadian men working primarily, though not exclusively, as independent escorts) combat the pervasive negativity that surrounds their profession. Semi-structured interviews were conducted with 9 men, a majority of whom were targeted through escort review boards. Interviews were transcribed verbatim and analysed for themes of "stigma resistance." Four themes were identified: (1) escorting is volitional (i.e., one isn't forced to work as an escort, rather it is a choice one makes); (2) escorting is a profession (i.e., the client is a customer and the escort a service provider); (3) the escort is in control during client/escort interchanges; and (4) escorting is distinct from, and better than, street prostitution. Directions for future research and limitations of the current study are outlined.

Todd G. Morrison is a lecturer at the National University of Ireland, Galway, Ireland. Bruce W. Whitehead is a sociology undergraduate student at the University of Calgary, Calgary, Alberta, Canada.

Address correspondence to: Dr. Todd G. Morrison, Department of Psychology, National University of Ireland, Galway, Ireland (E-mail: Todd.Morrison@nuigalway.ie).

The authors would like to thank the men who graciously agreed to be interviewed for this study.

[Haworth co-indexing entry note]: "Strategies of Stigma Resistance Among Canadian Gay-Identified Sex Workers." Morrison, Todd G., and Bruce W. Whitehead. Co-published simultaneously in *Journal of Psychology & Human Sexuality* (The Haworth Press, Inc.) Vol. 17, No. 1/2, 2005, pp. 169-179; and: *Contemporary Research on Sex Work* (ed: Jeffrey T. Parsons) The Haworth Press, Inc., 2005, pp. 169-179. Single or multiple copies of this article are available for a fee from The Haworth Document Delivery Service [1-800-HAWORTH, 9:00 a.m. - 5:00 p.m. (EST). E-mail address: docdelivery@haworthpress.com].

169

KEYWORDS. Prostitution, male prostitute, escort, sex industry, sex work, stigma, Canada

Minichiello and associates (2001) define sex work as any occupation where an individual is hired to provide sexual services in exchange for money and/or other items of value such as food, clothing, protection, and drugs. In accordance with this definition, the current study does not view sex work as an inherently degrading activity–one grounded in the subjugation of prostitute by client; rather, it is seen as a legitimate means of employment. This perspective does not assume that sex work ipso facto represents abjection of one's personhood nor does it preclude the occurrence of exploitation.

Although the topic of males employed in the sex industry has received some attention from social scientists, a majority of this research is HIV-related (Allman & Myers, 1999; Boles & Elifson, 1994; Elifson, Boles, & Sweat, 1993; Weinberg, Worth, & Williams, 2001) or concerned more globally with safer sex (Browne & Minichiello, 1995; Joffe & Dockrell, 1995; Marino, Browne, & Minichiello, 2000). Such research fails to particularize how these individuals, especially those that are gay-identified, interpret what they do within a social context that stigmatizes sex work. The issue of stigma (i.e., the branding of one's character that ensues from violating societal expectations) may be particularly salient among gay male sex workers because they embody two major taboos: homosexuality and prostitution (Koken, Bimbi, Parsons, & Halkitis, 2004).

The purpose of the current study was to examine ways in which gay-identified male sex workers may combat "society's ubiquitous cultural norms [surrounding prostitution]" (Scambler, 1997, p. 109)– norms stipulating that individuals working in this profession are "pathological" or "deviant" (Koken et al., 2004). Given Parsons, Bimbi, and Halkitis' (2001) concern that a majority of research focuses on one category of male sex worker (namely, street or bar hustlers), this study targeted escorts (i.e., sex workers who are self-employed and promote their services via gay media–primarily print and online).

METHOD

Participants

Nine male sex workers served as interviewees, with ages ranging from 20 to 42 ($M = 31.9$, $SD = 7.1$). Seven participants identified as Caucasian (or being of European heritage), one identified as Black, and one as being of mixed ethnicity. In terms of education, three of the participants had university degrees (2 undergraduate; 1 graduate); two were post-secondary students at the time the interviews were conducted; one had a partial university education; two had no post-secondary experience; and one had been trained (and employed) as a tradesman prior to becoming a sex worker.

Six of the men worked primarily in the sex industry whereas the other three also held "straight" jobs–two were professionals (e.g., financier) and one worked in a service sector position. As has been documented by other researchers (e.g., Minichiello et al., 2001), many participants engaged in more than one type of sex work such as adult film performer (both amateur and professional), escort, print model, brothel work, erotic dancer, domination/slave trainer, and erotic masseuse (2 men had received formal massage training).

Procedure

The three inclusion criteria for this study were that potential interviewees reside in Canada, identify as gay, and be self-employed. Therefore, men describing themselves as bisexual, advertising their services for women, claiming to be "gay for pay," working exclusively for an escort agency, and/or living outside of Canada were excluded.

An Internet search engine was used to locate sex worker review boards, which allow escorts both free and paid advertising and permit clients to access and post reviews of men and women in the sex industry. Internet links from the review boards and the sex workers' personal sites were used to locate additional prospective interviewees. Sites whose sole purpose was to advertise escorts also were investigated. Upon identifying potential participants, their e-mail addresses and primary locations (cities) of work were recorded. If the individual utilized a personal Website to advertise his services then that site was visited as well.

Five main sites (2 review boards and 3 escort lists) were instrumental in locating 118 potential participants. The men who were initially con-

sidered had personal e-mail addresses listed in their postings or advertisements. This criterion sought to eliminate agencies that advertised on
these sites and listed a number of sex workers (e.g., "worker's_name@
name_of_agency.com"). Recorded contact information was then
cross-referenced by city, name, identifying information (i.e., photos),
and e-mail address to ensure that men advertising under two or more
professional identities would not be subjected to duplicate contacts by
the researchers. Upon closer inspection, it was found that 43 of the 118
potential participants did not meet the study's inclusion criteria. Five
additional "persons" were duplicates of previously located participants
and, thus, were eliminated. Therefore, in the current study, 70
gay-identified male sex workers served as possible interviewees.

These individuals received an introductory letter via e-mail that explained the intent of the research, and information regarding the researchers and their intended use of the data. This letter stipulated clearly
that participation was voluntary and that all information gathered would
be anonymous and confidential. As well, prospective interviewees were
informed that they were "under no obligation to answer any of the questions posed during the interview [and] could withdraw from the study at
any point in time without penalty or consequence." Finally, the letter indicated that the study had been approved by a Human Research Ethics
Committee.

Of the 70 initial contacts, 10 e-mails were undeliverable. Forty-two
of the 60 e-mails received no acknowledgement; the remaining 18 provided a response. Two declined to participate and five offered to participate by e-mail correspondence only. Eleven men agreed to be
interviewed; however, 3 were unable to commit to an interview time
during the data collection period. Of the remaining 8, one recommended
another man for participation in the study. This individual agreed, resulting in 9 interviewees in total. Although the number of respondents is
small, it is congruent with other qualitative studies of male sex workers
(e.g., Browne & Minichiello, 1995, 1996).

Each of the nine interviewees received a copy of the consent form via
e-mail. As some interviews were conducted over the phone, a passive
consent procedure was used (i.e., verbal willingness to participate in the
study denoted acceptance of the terms and conditions outlined in the
consent form).

A semi-structured interview was conducted with participants being
asked a series of general questions followed by supplemental "trigger"
questions, if necessary. For example, each participant was asked, "Who
knows that you are employed in the sex industry?" In some cases, par-

ticipants provided considerable detail in response to this question. However, in other cases, follow-up items were needed such as "If you haven't told them, what do your family/friends think you do?" and "How do you decide whether or not to tell someone about what you do?" It should be noted that, although key topics were explored with all participants, variations in the interview schedule occurred. Indeed, participants determined large portions of interview content. It was believed that such flexibility would permit interviewees to disclose information that was most important to them.

The interviews ranged in length from approximately 60 minutes to three hours. They were tape-recorded and transcribed verbatim (i.e., paralinguistic cues such as "um" and "M-hmm" were included). One hundred eighty-seven pages of textual data were produced (single spaced, 12 point font).

These data were then evaluated using Interpretative Phenomenological Analysis (IPA), which is an analytic method well suited for small sample sizes (i.e., studies using IPA typically have 5 to 10 participants) (Smith, 2004). Stated briefly, IPA is "centred around exploring the experiences of individuals" (Shaw, 2001, p. 49) through in-depth examination of data collected using a qualitative methodology (typically, semi-structured interviews). Different levels of interpretation of textual data are possible; however, in all cases, interpretation must be grounded in the text itself. Consequently, "instead of attempting to support or refute an existing theory, researchers using IPA are able to investigate phenomena from a new perspective by learning from those who are *experiencing* [the phenomena]" (Shaw, 2001, p. 50, emphasis ours). In the current study, we were attempting to understand stigma resistance among gay male sex workers by interpreting the information they provided. We use the term "stigma resistance" rather than "stigma management" to denote a more active response to the negativity surrounding sex work in Western society. We regard the former as involving efforts to reconfigure those conditions engendering the stigma, and the latter as improving one's ability to function within the parameters of the stigma. From this perspective, techniques such as "passing" (i.e., keeping one's involvement as an escort secret from individuals other than one's clients–Koken et al., 2004) would be viewed as management rather than resistance. To reduce bias, we employed the strategy of researcher triangulation (Shaw, 2001) in which both authors reviewed the transcripts independently and then conferred to ensure that the themes identified were those which captured most accurately the collective voice of the interviewees.

RESULTS

Inspection of the transcripts suggests that participants used four main strategies to counteract the negativity surrounding their work in the sex industry. First, interviewees stressed the volitional nature of their involvement. None of the men in this study reported being coerced or forced into escort work; instead, the reasons underlying their decision to become escorts were multifarious.

> *. . . I was looking at it going. . . . Okay, I'm 20. I look pretty good, and I don't want to get to be 30 and then look back and go why did I . . . waste that? Why didn't I do that experience? I'm having the urge to . . . why hold back?* (Interviewee 4)

> *The first time I ever did it, I just wanted to know what the experience would be like. So, I met someone who was doing it. I didn't seek him out, but I just happened to meet this guy, and I asked him if . . . he ever needed another person to come with him to let me know.* (Interviewee 5)

> *I was here in Canada from [country omitted] and I needed money, so . . . I was thinking [about escorting] for a while and I decided to put an ad in the paper and see . . . how it would go.* (Interviewee 6)

> *My current boyfriend . . . had been doing it before I met him. So, that's how . . . the idea . . . got in my head. And . . . it was beneficial to me to be able to talk to people who had been doing it before . . . to try and give me a heads up about what it was all about.* (Interviewee 1)

Without exception, participants also reported that, if they wished to, they could leave the sex industry at any time.

Second, interviewees stressed that, when interacting with a customer, they were the ones in control.

> *I'm in control of the situation. I don't do anything that I'm uncomfortable with . . . that I think might be dangerous for me.* (Interviewee 1)

> *By default the escort has the control. No doubt about it. The escort only loses the control when they give it up.* (Interviewee 3)

[In response to a question concerning whether the customer or client is in control] *It's me. It has to be me. . . . The guy's pretty scared. You have to be gentle with him and make him feel comfortable. That's the first job. So, that's all the control.* (Interviewee 6)

According to participants, this control also manifested itself in terms of what they were willing to do sexually with a client.

I don't do stuff I don't want to do . . . but . . . that's why you've got to talk to your clients before you even, like, go see them. (Interviewee 8)

I'm just like, you know what, absolutely not . . . I will not do it. They're like "well, what are you in this for?" Like, not for that. If you want somebody for that then you go and find somebody for that. (Interviewee 9)

The third method of stigma resistance that was evident in the transcripts was interviewees' perception of escorts as professionals.

I have an MBA (Master's in Business Administration). I mean I am not . . . some punk off the street. But even if I didn't actually have a degree to my name. . . . I am a professional person. My career is not the same as their career, but nonetheless I am a professional person. I do demand respect from all my clients and I do mean demand. (Interviewee 3)

I took the time. I read books. I read everything. I met people who were doing it [escorting]. I watched how they answered their phones. [And] then [I] developed my own routine around it. (Interviewee 4)

This perception of "escort as professional" also was evident in the language participants used to describe what they do for a living. They employed terminology such as "volume of clients," and described escorting as a "business" and an "industry." Some interviewees spoke of "marketing" and "promoting" their services, and referred to their involvement in other aspects of the sex industry (e.g., pornography) as "infomercials" for their escort work.

The fourth, and final, technique concerned the boundaries participants established between various forms of sex work; primarily the distinction between escort worker and street prostitute.

> *The difference for me [is] you're a hooker . . . you work for drugs.*
> *[With] escorts . . . it's a little more . . . maybe a little class . . . you*
> *don't have to stand on the corner of the street. I think if I [were] a*
> *street prostitute, I would have no respect. Zero. Absolutely none.*
> (Interviewee 9).

> *I mean I've got a university degree. I have a career with a finan-*
> *cial company. I've been with a partner for almost three years. . . .*
> *I've got a pretty good lifestyle and I think people need to realize*
> *that it's not just, you know, some drug addict runaway or whatever*
> *that's out there selling a blowjob for 20 bucks.* (Interviewee 1)

Although the distinction between escort and street prostitute often
centred on personal agency (or lack thereof), participants also differentiated between the two on the basis of price.

> *I think there's respect for the upper end of the scale. I mean my*
> *half-sister, who's 19 . . . [when she found out] . . . one of her ques-*
> *tions at one point was "Um, are you expensive?" So, there's this*
> *idea that, well, if you're expensive then . . . that's OK, that's good.*
> (Interviewee 5)

> *. . . If I see that they're just charging 100 bucks an hour, I know*
> *they're doing it for the wrong reason.* (Interviewee 8)

> *I am the highest priced masseur in [city omitted]. Hands down.*
> *Period. You get what you pay for.* (Interviewee 3)

DISCUSSION

These findings suggest that the male sex workers in this study appeared to use four principal "strategies of resistance" in response to the
hegemonic discourse surrounding those employed in the sex industry–a
discourse that characterises these individuals as pathological and deviant. Participants: (a) emphasized the volitional nature of escorting;
(b) asserted that they were in control during client/escort encounters;

(c) evaluated what they did through a lens of professionalism; and (d) maintained firm demarcations between various categories of sex work (in particular, the distinction between escorting and street prostitution).

In a recent study examining stigma management among American gay male escorts, Koken et al. (2004) similarly found that some participants used an "entrepreneurial framework" as a means of coping with the negativity surrounding the sex industry. However, other management techniques identified by these authors (which similarly might be viewed as forms of resistance) did not emerge as predominant themes in our transcripts. For example, we did not find that interviewees regarded sex work as analogous to a "helping profession" such as psychotherapy or nursing.

Interestingly, a key component of the strategies of resistance identified in the current study appears to be denigration of street prostitutes, who in comparison to escorts (purportedly) lack volition; are dependent on the client; have "no professional product" to sell; and occupy the lowest stratum of the sex work hierarchy. It is ironic that interviewees' perceptions of street prostitutes (or hustlers) reflect many of the negative stereotypes mainstream culture possesses about the sex industry in general. An important question for future research is why did participants evidence this factionalism? Do they believe that greater acceptance of one category of sex worker is contingent upon greater derogation of another category? Why didn't participants generate "strategies of resistance" designed to challenge predominant views of the sex industry overall rather than escorts in particular?

As with any study, there are limitations that warrant mention. First, although the sample appeared to be fairly heterogeneous in terms of age, geographic location, and services provided, the number of participants used was small. Second, self-selection bias is a concern. Obviously those agreeing to participate in this study may have had greater interest in the topics under discussion. As one participant remarked:

> *That's why I wanted to do this interview cause I was like, you know, I'm not living in a box. . . . I'm not some freak or something.*
> (Interviewee 8)

Those with similar motivations may be overrepresented in the current sample and, thus, may provide a distorted view of the experiences of "higher end" sex workers.

An additional limitation concerns the veracity of participants' self-disclosure. To reduce self-presentational concerns, the authors emphasized the importance of honesty in their consent protocol and made it clear that their motivation was to collect, rather than judge, sex workers' experiences. The similarity in themes identified across participants, living in different regions of Canada, reduced the authors' concerns about the "validity" issue. However, it is certainly possible that interviewees may have fabricated some or all of the information they disclosed. If interviewees' motivation was to "prove" they are "normal" (e.g., Interviewee 8), they might have used information strategically to convey that impression.

In summary, it appears that some gay-identified male sex workers may challenge society's view of sex work, as it pertains to escorting, through a variety of resistance techniques. Such findings underscore the need to move beyond narrow avenues of inquiry (e.g., sex worker as vector of HIV/AIDS transmission) and to avoid reductionistic and irresolvable issues affiliated with the prostitution is good/prostitution is bad debate.

REFERENCES

Allman, D., & Myers, T. (1999). Male sex work and HIV/AIDS in Canada. In P. Aggleton (Ed.), *Men who sell sex: International perspectives on male prostitution and HIV/AIDS* (pp. 61-81). Philadelphia: Temple University Press.

Boles, J., & Elifson, K.W. (1994). Sexual identity and HIV: The male prostitute. *The Journal of Sex Research, 31*, 39-46.

Browne, J., & Minichiello, V. (1995). The social meanings behind male sex work: Implications for sexual interactions. *British Journal of Sociology, 46*, 598-622.

Browne, J., & Minichiello, V. (1996). The social and work context of commercial sex between men: A research note. *Australian and New Zealand Journal of Sociology, 32*, 86-92.

Elifson, K.W., Boles, J., & Sweat, M. (1993). Risk factors associated with HIV infection among male prostitutes. *American Journal of Public Health, 83*, 79-83.

Joffe, H., & Dockrell, J.E. (1995). Safer sex: Lessons from the male sex industry. *Journal of Community & Applied Social Psychology, 5*, 333-346.

Koken, J.A., Bimbi, D.S., Parsons, J.T., & Halkitis, P.N. (2004). The experience of stigma in the lives of male Internet escorts. *Journal of Psychology and Human Sexuality, 16*(1), 13-32.

Marino, R., Browne, J., & Minichiello, V. (2000). An instrument to measure safer sex strategies used by male sex workers. *Archives of Sexual Behavior, 29*, 217-228.

Minichiello, V., Marino, R., Browne, J., Jamieson, M., Peterson, K., Reuter, B., & Robinson, K. (2001). Male sex workers in three Australian cities: Socio-demographic and sex work characteristics. *Journal of Homosexuality, 42*, 29-51.

Parsons, J.T., Bimbi, D., & Halkitis, P.N. (2001). Sexual compulsivity among gay/bisexual male escorts who advertise on the Internet. *Sexual Addiction & Compulsivity, 8*, 101-112.

Scambler, G. (1997). Conspicuous and inconspicuous sex work: The neglect of the ordinary and mundane. In G. Scambler & A. Scambler (Eds.), *Rethinking prostitution: Purchasing sex in the 1990s* (pp. 105-120). New York: Routledge.

Shaw, R. (2001). Why use interpretative phenomenological analysis in health psychology? *Health Psychology Update, 10*(4), 48-52.

Smith, J.A. (2004). Reflecting on the development of interpretative phenomenological analysis and its contribution to qualitative research in psychology. *Qualitative Research in Psychology, 1*, 39-54.

Weinberg, M.S., Worth, H., & Williams, C.J. (2001). Men sex workers and other men who have sex with men: How do their HIV risks compare in New Zealand? *Archives of Sexual Behaviour, 30*, 273-286.

Self-Reported Use of Health Services, Contact with Police and Views About Sex Work Organizations Among Male Sex Workers in Cordoba, Argentina

Carlos E. Disogra, PhD(c)
Rodrigo Mariño, PhD
Victor Minichiello, PhD

SUMMARY. A total of 31 male sex workers recruited in Cordoba, Argentina, completed a questionnaire about the use and barriers to the use

---

Carlos E. Disogra is affiliated with the Faculty of Psychology, Universidad Nacional de Cordoba, Cordoba, Argentina, and is currently completing his PhD studies.

Rodrigo Mariño and Victor Minichiello are affiliated with the School of Health, University of New England, Armidale, New South Wales, Australia.

Address correspondence to: Victor Minichiello, School of Health, University of New England, Armidale, New South Wales, Australia 2350 (E-mail: vminichi@pobox.une.edu.au).

The authors would like to thank the participants in this study, in particular Dr. Eduardo Cosacov for supporting the project and Dr. Robin Lin Miller and Nadine Stevoff for assisting with identifying key references for this study.

This study was funded by grants from the Australian Research Council (ARC) in Australia and the Secretary of Science and Technology of the Universidad Nacional de Cordoba, Argentina.

[Haworth co-indexing entry note]: "Self-Reported Use of Health Services, Contact with Police and Views About Sex Work Organizations Among Male Sex Workers in Cordoba, Argentina." Disogra, Carlos E., Rodrigo Mariño, and Victor Minichiello. Co-published simultaneously in *Journal of Psychology & Human Sexuality* (The Haworth Press, Inc.) Vol. 17, No. 1/2, 2005, pp. 181-195; and: *Contemporary Research on Sex Work* (ed: Jeffrey T. Parsons) The Haworth Press, Inc., 2005, pp. 181-195. Single or multiple copies of this article are available for a fee from The Haworth Document Delivery Service [1-800-HAWORTH, 9:00 a.m. - 5:00 p.m. (EST). E-mail address: docdelivery@haworthpress.com].

of health services, contact with the police and perception about the need of sex workers organizations. The results reveal that the majority preferred to use public services for general and sexual health concerns. The most frequently identified barriers to use of health services were waiting time before consultation and opening hours. The majority agreed for the need of a sex workers organization to advocate on their behalf, particularly achieving decriminalization of sex work and providing sexual health information to sex workers. Many reported contact with police that was generally positive, although some concerns were raised. The paper discusses implications for public health measures aimed at promoting greater sexual safety in the male sex industry. *[Article copies available for a fee from The Haworth Document Delivery Service: 1-800-HAWORTH. E-mail address: <docdelivery@haworthpress.com> Website: <http://www.HaworthPress.com> © 2005 by The Haworth Press, Inc. All rights reserved.]*

KEYWORDS. Male sex work, health services, community organizations, police, Argentina

The published literature on male sex workers (MSWs) can be organized as pre- and post-HIV/AIDS and reveals significantly different research focuses and frameworks (Browne & Minichiello, 1996). In the pre-HIV/AIDS period the attention was on the "individual" worker with the objective to explore the causes of the behavior that was generally viewed as a deviant activity (Ginsburg, 1967; Coombs, 1974; Caukins & Coombs, 1976; Allen, 1980; Earls & David, 1989). Up until the past decades, few studies analyzed male sex work for its public health significance, as a hospitality occupation, or for gaining a wider conceptual understanding of male-to-male sexuality or masculinity. A homophobic attitude and criminology perspective generally underpinned the topic (Browne & Minichiello, 1997); however, this has now been challenged as researchers have studied aspects of the sex industry as a form of work/occupation and commenced to deconstruct the deviant and illegal discourses (Scott, Minichiello, Mariño, Harvey & Jamieson, 2005; Minichiello, Mariño, Browne & Jamieson, 1998).

The HIV/AIDS epidemic marked the beginning of a new focus for research. Studies centered on the behavior and sexual practices that increased safer sex outcomes and minimized the spread of HIV and sexually transmitted infections (STIs) in the community and sex industry. Large-scale surveys on MSWs, and to a lesser extent on their clients, have been conducted in Australia (Minichiello et al., 1999; 2001; Minichiello, Mariño, Browne & Jamieson, 2000; Estcourt et al., 2000); Brazil (Cortes et al., 1989), Canada (Weber et al., 2001), the United States of America (Elifson, Boles & Sweat, 1993; Simon, Morse, Blazon, Osofsky & Gaumer, 1993), the United Kingdom (West & de Villiers, 1993), Thailand (Kunawararak et al., 1995), the Netherlands (Coutinho, van Andel & Rijsdijk, 1988), Spain (Belza et al., 2001), New Zealand (Weinberg, Worth & Williams, 2001), Thailand (Kunawararak et al., 1995) and Indonesia (Ford, Wirawan, Fajans & Thorpe, 1995). By the end of the century effective HIV and STI prevention interventions in the sex industry were reported in the United States (Miller, Klotz & Eckholdt, 1998) and the United Kingdom (Ziersch, Gaffney & Tomlinson, 2000). Yet despite these successes and the call from researchers to develop comprehensive social and health services particularly designed for MSWs, there is not, for instance, widespread support for establishing these services. It is encouraging to see, however, the emergence of support groups such as the European Network Male Prostitution (ENMP) that disseminates information about the development of health and education strategies and services to MSWs (www.enmp.org).

The study of health service utilization by MSWs is almost nonexistent. Only one study was found reporting on health service utilization by MSWs. Snell (1991) found that over half of his MSWs indicated that they would, for example, seek help from hospital emergency wards, medical clinics, ministers or lawyers, and 39% would seek help from a social service or welfare agency, mental health centre, or private therapists. The majority indicated that they were satisfied with the help they received from such formal services, and 91% indicated that would return to the same person or place for further assistance. The fact that men generally use health and social services less frequently than women (Addis & Mahalik, 2003) emphasizes the need to better understand the barriers associated with accessing such services. Yet no one can deny that regular contact with health services provides opportunities for early diagnosis and treatment of disease and for maintenance of a good health status. More importantly, they provide the forum for sexual health promotion, sexual health education and prevention through behavioral changes.

Argentina is a federal republic with a population of 36 million people. Cordoba is the second largest city with a population of 1.3 million. Although there are several organizations concerned with the prevention of the HIV transmission in Argentina, and a female sex workers union operates in Buenos Aires, Argentina does not have any specific public services funded by the state with a mandate to, for example, offer services to sex workers or run specific health promotion or peer education programs. Health promotion and education programs are by and large run by volunteers at a local level. These include human rights groups and sporadic and short-lived gay organizations.

The importance of such public organizations is that they serve two roles: to communicate with and offer support to the sex worker community. In so doing, they provide an important function in liaising and communicating with government bodies, community groups and the criminal justice system, and offering a range of health and social support, health education and information programs to sex workers. Although there has not been a systematic evaluation about the social and health effects of these organizations on the sex industry, they have a clear public health role and are highly regarded by sex workers. For example, a research conducted in Australia found that MSWs' contact with sex workers organizations and sexual health clinics may play an important role in helping them to adopt public health strategies that result in client compliance with safer sex (Mariño, Minichiello, Browne, 2000).

Prostitution is legal in Argentina. However, in Cordoba offering sex services on the street is an offence carrying a sentence of up to 20 days of imprisonment, but this regulation is not always enforced by the police. Yet police attitudes and behaviors may have important public health implications, including in Argentina and other countries such as the United Kingdom and Sri Lanka, where there are reports of the police searching for condoms on MSWs, removing them, making negative comments about the worker, or using condoms as evidence of working as a sex worker (West & Villiers, 1993; Ratnapala, 1999). This goes against public interest as it may prevent safer sex behaviors. However, the police might be encouraged to play a partnership role in curbing the HIV infection. For example, investigators in Sri Lanka visited the police and distributed condoms to them with the intention that they assist with its distribution (Ratnapala, 1999).

If safer sex and healthier choices and accessing appropriate services are to be encouraged and maintained among MSWs, and in the absence of specific studies on MSMs on this topic, it is important to investigate the use of health and social services by MSWs and to identify perceived barriers to use such services. This exploratory study was undertaken, firstly, to describe whether male sex workers in Cordoba use health services and their level of satisfaction with them; secondly, to identify self-reported barriers to use these services; and thirdly, to examine factors associated with use of health services. Additionally, due to the implications with safe sex behaviors and for the design of future interventions among MSWs, it was also considered important to investigate contact with the police and the MSWs' perception of the need and role of sex workers organizations.

METHODS

Participants and Procedure

With the approval from the Ethics and Research Committee of University of New England and fulfillment of the ethics requirements from the Faculty of Psychology of the National University of Cordoba, MSWs from Cordoba who were men and dressed as men, aged 18 years and older and currently selling their sexual services to other men were invited to participate in the study. After an MSW gave written consent to participate in the project, he was asked to complete and return a questionnaire, and to contact the field coordinator to arrange a convenient time to discuss instructions on how to complete other study instruments. The characteristics of the sample and research methodology used are described in detail elsewhere (Mariño, Minichiello & Disogra, 2003; Mariño, Minichiello & Disogra, 2004).

Different sampling strategies were used to recruit participants in the different modalities. For independent male sex workers (IMSWs), a list of potential participants was compiled by reviewing the local media where IMSWs advertise. For street workers (SMSWs), convenience samples were recruited from locations where such workers sell their services to clients.

Measures

The questionnaire included personal and sex work characteristics and previously validated scales on knowledge about safer sex, attitudes to condom use and HIV/STIs risk perceptions (Minichiello et al., 1999; Mariño et al., 2000; Mariño et al., 2003). The final section of the questionnaire covered MSWs' use of health and social services. Participants were asked about their perceived need for a sex workers association and about their contact with the police.

Participants were given a list of alternative places of treatment for both general and sexual illnesses, and were asked to indicate their preference of treatment sites, access and, when they had used the services, the perceived rating of the service received. Regarding use of general/sexual health services, participants were asked to indicate, from a list of ten alternatives, where they generally went when they felt ill or were concerned that they had a sexual infection. These included: public hospital, private hospital, health assistance centre, private GP, a chemist, other MSW, friends, relatives, a healer or nobody. A second question asked participants to rate on a five-point ordinal scale the perceived quality of the services, ranging from *Excellent* to *Bad*.

Participants were asked, from a list of five commonly described categories, about self-perceived barriers to general/sexual health care service utilization. Categories included: opening times, time waiting for attention, rude behavior from health service staff, location of services, and cost. Additionally, MSWs were asked whether they avoided using health services for either general health problems or sexual health problems.

Another set of questions asked about the perceived need for sex workers organizations in Cordoba. Participants were also asked from a list of 11 activities to indicate the type of activities that such an organization could do on behalf of MSWs. The activities were to: stop prejudices against sex workers; stop discrimination against sex workers; achieve decriminalization of sex work; provide legal information to sex workers; provide advice on alternative sources of jobs for those who want to change occupation; provide sexual health information to sex workers; provide safe sex supplies at lower prices; distribute free condoms; organize vaccination campaigns for sex workers; keep a list of violent clients; and organize social gatherings for sex workers.

MSWs were asked whether they had contact with the police while working as a sex worker. Those who had contact were asked about the frequency of these contacts. Finally, MSWs were asked about the outcome of the contact (i.e., physical or verbal violence, sexual abuse, detention, asked for money, asked you to leave the area, or asked for free sexual services).

Data Analysis

Results are analyzed in two ways. Firstly, basic descriptive information on the distribution of the main variables by sex work modality (e.g., street or independent), and secondly, chi-square or t-test analysis to evaluate the relationship of modality of work with categorical data and ordinal data and continuous variables, respectively. However, in some cases, since only a small number of MSWs appeared in some of the categories, no further statistical comparisons could be performed. Data manipulation and analyses were done using SPSS PC (version 9.0) (Nourisis, 1998).

RESULTS

Data collection occurred from mid-January 2001 to mid-December 2001. A total of 47 MSWs were contacted. Thirty-five agreed to participate and complete the questionnaire, representing a response rate of 74.5%. However, three participants were younger than the age criteria and another was eliminated because he indicated working in the male-to-female sex industry only. Of the remaining 31, 17 of them worked as SMSWs and 14 as IMSWs. Although a difficult population to develop reliable sample population figures, it is estimated as a result of discussions with police and other authorities that this sample captures between more than one-third and less than half of the MSW population working in the city at the time of the study.

The age of MSWs ranged from 18 to 37 years old (Mean = 25.1; SD = 5.93). By modality of work, SMSWs were significantly younger (Mean = 21.7) than IMSWs (Mean = 29.3) (t(29) = 20.82, p < .001). With regards to education level, 45.2% of the MSWs overall had completed at least secondary education. By type of work, IMSWs had completed significantly higher levels of education than SMSWs. For example, 57.1% of the IMSWs had some level of tertiary education compared to 11.8% of SMSWs ($\chi^2(1)$ = 7.24, p < .01).

A majority of the MSWs were renting accommodation (with flatmates or alone) or living with their parents (38.7%, and 32.3%, respectively), with the rest owning their own place, or having other living arrangements. IMSWs were more likely to live independently in rented place (64.3%) than SMSW (17.7%), while SMSWs were more likely to live with their parents (52.9% vs. 7.1%) (($\chi^2(2)$ = 9.31, p < .01). When describing their sexual identity, the most frequent answer was "heterosexual (straight)" (33.3%), closely followed by "gay" (30%). Twenty percent described themselves as "bisexual," and 16.7% indicated other sexual orientations.

The most frequent period working as a sex worker was 2 to 5 years. By modality of work, IMSWs tended to have been working longer in the sex industry. For example, 57.1% of the IMSWs had worked in the industry for more than 2 years, compared to 41.1% of the SMSWs.

Access to Health Care Services

Regarding use of health services, the majority mentioned that the preferred place for consultation for both general and sexual health concerns was the public hospital (67.7% and 60%, respectively). In the case of general health concerns, the second and third preferred places were the health assistance centre (16.1%) and private hospital (12.9%). Regarding sexual health concerns, the second most frequently nominated place was a friend (23.3%), followed by private hospital (16.7%), the health assistance centre (16.1%), and relatives (10%). None of the other alternatives reached 10% for either general or sexual health problems.

Beliefs About Health Care Services

As Table 1 reveals the three most frequent barriers to use health care services were: the length of waiting time, opening time and the cost of services in that order.

The majority of participants (54.8%) reported one barrier to accessing general health care services; 29.0% and 9.7% reported two or more than two barriers, respectively, and the remainder 6.5% reported no barriers. Regarding sexual health care services, the largest group (48.4%)

TABLE 1. Self-Perceived Barriers to General/Sexual Health Care Service Utilization

Barriers[a]	General health %[b]	Sexual health %[c]
Time waiting for attention	82.1	70.4
Opening times	41.4	33.3
Cost of services	24.1	22.2
Rude behavior from health professionals	17.2	14.8
Location of services	10.3	11.1

[a]Note. Participants could nominate more than one barrier.
[b]n = 27.
[c]n = 29.

reported one barrier; 19.4% and 13% reported two and three or four conditions, respectively, and 19.4% reported no barriers. Number of barriers was recoded into three groups (no barriers, one barrier, two barriers or more barriers) for further analyses. No significant differences by type of sex work were found in relation to barriers to use health care services.

When rating health services, participants considered consultations for sexual health concerns to be better than for general health. About 42% rated general health consultations as ordinary, or bad, compared to only 28.5% for sexual health consultations. The majority rated sexual health services as good or very good (53.6%), while only 45.2% rated general health services in that way. The remainder rated general/sexual health services as excellent.

About half of the respondents indicated that they avoided the use of general health services (n = 15), but few reported having avoided sexual health services (n = 2) for any reason. There were no differences by modality of sex work. Reasons for avoiding were also explored; however, sample sizes limitations precluded any conclusion on this topic.

Sex Workers Advocacy

The great majority (67.7%) responded that there should be a sex worker organization in Cordoba. As shown in Table 2, among those who support the need for such an organization (n = 23), the most mentioned activities for the organization were: complete decriminalization of sex work, and provision of sexual health information (65.2% each); provision of job alternative for those willing to leave sex work (60.9%); work to stop prejudices against sex workers; and organization of vaccination campaigns for sex workers (52.2% each). Most participants (81%) agreed with at least two activities, while 57.1% nominated six or more of the activities. There were significant differences on the expected activities according to modality of sex work; IMSWs were more likely than SMSWs to support the following activities: provision of legal information to MSWs (25% vs. 72.7%; ($\chi^2(1) = 5.24$, $p < .05$), and organizing a health insurance for MSWs (8.3% vs. 63.6%; ($\chi^2(1) = 7.74$, $p < .01$).

Contacts with the Police

As shown in Table 3, more than half (54.8%) of the respondents had contact with the police while working as sex workers. SMSWs had sig-

TABLE 2. Proportion of Participants Who Nominated Each of the Activities That a Sex Workers Organization Could Do on Behalf of MSW

Activity[a]	%[b]
To achieve complete decriminalization of sex work	65.2
To provide sexual health information to sex workers	65.2
To advise on alternative sources of jobs for those who want to change occupation	60.9
To stop prejudices against sex workers	52.2
To organize vaccination campaigns for sex workers	52.2
To provide legal information to sex workers	47.8
To provide safe sex supplies at lower prices	47.8
To stop discrimination against sex workers	43.5
To organize social gatherings for sex workers	43.5
To distribute free condoms	39.1
To organize a health insurance for sex workers	34.8
To keep a list of violent clients	30.4
To advise boys who want to begin working as sex workers	21.7
Others	4.5

[a] *Note.* Participants could nominate more than one activity.
[b] $n = 23$.

nificantly more frequent contact with the police (82.4% vs. 21.4%; ($\chi^2(1) = 11.51, p < .001$). Of those SMSWs and IMSWs who indicated contact with the police, the frequencies of such contacts were: most of the time or almost all the time (17.7%); for 35.3% of the respondents these contacts were only occasional; and for 47.0% they were very rare. However, IMSWs reported that they had occasional or very rare contacts with the police. Independent of the frequency of these contacts, police asked the sex workers to leave the area (70.6%) or took them to the police station (23.5%). On very few occasions were the police physically violent (11.8%) or verbally abusive (11.8%). On the other hand, in 23.5% of the cases, it was reported that the police acted professionally. Three participants indicated that the police checked for condoms, but none indicated that the possession of condoms was used as evidence that they were working as a sex worker.

TABLE 3. Reported Contacts Between MSW and the Police and Police's Attitude During the Contact

Contact	%[a]
No	45.2
Yes	54.8
Police attitudes during the contact[b, c]	
Officers asked MSW to leave the area	70.6
Officers took the MSW to the station	23.5
Officers acted professionally	23.5
Officers physically violent	11.8
Officers verbally abusive	11.8
Officers verified whether the MSW had condoms	17.7

[a]*Note. n = 30*
[b]Participants could nominate more than one alternative.
[c]*n = 17*. Only those who reported contact with the police

DISCUSSION

The findings of this study are derived from a small sample of MSWs recruited in Cordoba from two modalities of sex work. One agency advertising male-to-male commercial sex was found through the local media. Attempts were made to recruit MSWs working in agencies, but this proved unsuccessful. Although the results should be interpreted within the restraints and limitations imposed by sample size, it captured a high proportion of the MSW population from Cordoba. Interestingly, the sample size obtained in the present study is not different from that obtained in a city of similar size (Brisbane, Australia) by Minichiello and his collaborators (2001). Thus, this paper represents a preliminary insight to better understanding some of the issues associated with the use of health services by MSWs, a largely unexamined area of research. The result could provide policy makers and practitioners with information that may assist in the design of health and sexual health promotion and risk minimization programs, and ensuring that interventions are properly designed to address the needs of the MSW groups. For example, most participants reported the preference to receive general health and sexual health treatment from a public hospital. Health care professionals working in this area are in a key position to contact MSWs and should be aware of this situation by, for example, reinforcing educational messages, but above all, avoiding unnecessary questions (do you work as a sex worker?), assuring confidentiality, and other sensitive issues when working with at-risk and marginalized groups who otherwise could have little access to vital health information.

It was also found that MSWs prefer to receive sexual health consultation and treatment from friends. This would suggest that peer and community education might be relevant for sexual issues, perhaps developing "mentoring" or role model programs. Such an activity could be the responsibility of, for example, an MSW organization that employs previous MSWs as outreach community workers to provide peer support and education and serve as role models. This very model has proved to be very successful in Australia, where state governments have established and funded sex work organizations and the services are highly used by sex workers (Browne & Minichiello, 1997). Likewise, the Working Men Project in the United Kingdom is another example where peer support is offered to encourage MSWs to maintain good sexual health (see www.wmplondon.org.uk). Additionally, interventions in this group may start by promoting a positive image of sexual health clinics as a source of information. Understanding the benefits of using health services may help to overcome perceived barriers. Further studies may also aim to clarify whether cultural difference between health professionals and sex workers (due to age, homophobia or sexual orientation) affects this relationship.

General and sexual health services may not have been accessed for many reasons. Access to clinical services faces many financial and structural barriers as well as attitudinal factors among both users and providers. Therefore, while increasing efforts should be directed to addressing structural barriers, such as length of waiting time before treatment and opening hours, there is an additional need to address the full range of the users' barriers and concerns. Failure to address this issue is likely to create obstacles, and policy initiatives might fail, not because of lack of research about MSWs health behaviors, but because of structural factors that do not allow certain outcomes to be realistically achieved.

Contacts between the police and MSWs were infrequent, particularly, and not unexpectedly, among IMSWs. In the majority of cases where there was a contact, police appeared to have acted professionally and most frequently MSWs reported that they were not arrested but asked to leave the area. There were no cases of alleged rape and when the police detected condoms it was not used as evidence to charge for sex work. These reported behaviors are to be highly praised and encouraged. On the other hand, a few MSWs self-reported being the victim of physical violence from the police. Although a small number, this represents a significant issue that needs further study. Innovative methods, such as the one adopted in Sri Lanka (Ratnapala, 1999), might enhance the ability of police to influence high-risk sexual behaviors. Furthermore, it might turn checking MSWs for condoms into a safer-sex campaign rather than a criminal surveillance.

In the present study, MSWs clearly appreciated the benefits of a sex workers organization that provide services for them. Elsewhere, the use of sex work organizations has been instrumental in achieving effective regulation of the sex industry and providing sexual health information and other services to sex workers (e.g., Sex Workers Outreach Project, 2003). Differences in the support and perhaps willingness to use such service according to modality of sex work must be noted. MSWs who do not self-identify as gay or see themselves as part of the gay community might not access the services of such organizations if they are closely aligned with the gay community (Mariño et al., 2003). However, there is evidence to suggest that these organizations have successfully established close ties and trust with MSWs, and isolated MSWs in particular, as well as with escort agencies' owners or managers. Future research needs to explore the impact of such organizations on the public perception of the sex industry, and what benefits they provide in terms of promoting a more professional and safer service and enhancing the self-esteem of the sex worker as a professional operating in a more regulated hospitality industry. We also recommend that a larger national study in Argentina of the male sex industry, with possible comparisons with the female sex industry, is now warranted. In addition, some qualitative studies that focus on how non-gay identifying MSWs make sense of their experiences in general and specifically with clients, the police and health professionals would shed further knowledge on this topic.

REFERENCES

Addis, M. E., & Mahalik, J. R. (2003). Men, masculinity, and the contexts of help seeking. *American Psychologist, 58*, 5-14.

Allen, D. M. (1980). Young male prostitutes: A psychosocial study. *Archives of Sexual Behavior, 9*, 399-426.

Belza, M. J., Llacer, A., Mora, R., Morales, M., Castilla, J., & de la Fuente, L. (2001). Socio-demographic characteristics and HIV behavior patterns of male sex workers in Madrid, Spain. *AIDS Care, 13*, 677-682.

Browne, J., & Minichiello, V. (1996). Research directions in male sex work. *Journal of Homosexuality, 31*, 29-56.

Browne, J., & Minichiello, V. (1997). Promoting safer sex in the male sex work industry: A professional responsibility. *AIDS Patient Care and STDs, 11*, 353-358.

Caukins, S. E., & Coombs, N. R. (1976). The psychodynamics of male prostitution. *American Journal of Psychotherapy, 30*, 441-451.

Coombs, N. R. (1974). Male prostitution: A psychological view of behavior. *American Journal of Orthopsychiatry, 44*, 782-789.

Cortes, E., Detels, R., Aboulafia, D., Li, X., Moudgil, T., Alam, M., Bonecker, C., Gonzaga, A., Oyafuzo, F., Tondo, M., Boite, C., Hammershlak, N., Capitani, C., Slamon, D., & Ho, D. (1989). HIV-1, HIV-2, and HTLV-1 infection in high-risk groups in Brazil. *New England Journal of Medicine, 320*, 953-958.

Coutinho, R. A., van Andel, R. L. M., & Rijsdijk, T. J. (1988). Role of male prostitutes in spread of sexually transmitted diseases and human immunodeficiency virus. *Genitourinary Medicine, 64*, 207-208.

Earls, C. M., & David, H. (1989). A psychosocial study of male prostitution. *Archives of Sexual Behavior, 18*, 401-419.

Elifson, K. W., Boles, J., & Sweat, M. (1993). Risk factors associated with HIV infection among male prostitutes. *American Journal of Public Health, 83*, 79-83.

Estcourt, C. S., Marks, C., Rohrsheim, R., Johnson, A. M., Donovan, B., & Mindel, A. (2000). HIV, sexually transmitted infections, and risk behaviors in male commercial sex workers in Sydney. *Sexually Transmitted Infections, 76*, 294-308.

Ford, K., Wirawan, D. N., Fajans, P., & Thorpe, L. (1995). AIDS knowledge, risk behaviors, and factors related to condom use among male commercial sex workers and male tourist clients in Bali, Indonesia. *AIDS, 9*, 751-759.

Ginsburg, K. N. (1967). The "meat-rack": A study of the male homosexual prostitute. *American Journal of Psychotherapy, 21*, 170-185.

Kunawararak, P., Beyrer, C., Natpratan, C., Feng, W., Celentano, D. D., de Boer, M., Nelson, K. E., & Khamboonruang, C. (1995). The epidemiology of HIV and syphilis among male commercial sex workers in northern Thailand. *AIDS, 9*, 517-521.

Mariño, R., Browne, J., & Minichiello, V. (2000). An instrument to measure safer sex strategies used by male sex workers. *Archives of Sexual Behavior, 29*, 217-228.

Mariño, R., Minichiello, V., & Disogra, C. (2003). Male sex workers in Cordoba, Argentina: Socio-demographic characteristics and sex work experiences. *Pan American Journal of Public Health, 13*, 311-319.

Mariño, R., Minichiello, V., & Disogra, C. (2004). A profile of clients of male sex workers in Cordoba, Argentina. *International Journal of STD & AIDS, 15*, 266-272.

Miller, R. L., Klotz, D., & Eckholdt, H. M. (1998). HIV prevention with male prostitutes and patrons of hustler bars: Replication of an HIV preventive intervention. *American Journal of Community Psychology, 26*, 97-131.

Minichiello, V., Marino, R., Khan, A., & Browne, J. (2003). Alcohol and drug use in Australian male sex workers: its relationship to the safety outcome of the sex encounter. *AIDS Care, 15*, 549-562.

Minichiello, V., Mariño, R., & Browne, J. (2001). Knowledge, risk perceptions and condom usage in male sex workers from three Australian cities. *AIDS Care, 13*, 387-402.

Minichiello, V., Mariño, R., Browne, J., Jamieson, M., Peterson, K., Reuter, B., & Robinson, K. (1999). A profile of the clients of male sex workers in three Australian cities. *Australian and New Zealand Journal of Public Health, 23*(5), 511-518.

Minichiello, V., Mariño, R., Browne, J., Jamieson, M., Peterson, K., Reuter, B., & Robinson, K. (2001). Male sex workers in three Australian cities: Socio-demographic and sex work characteristics. *Journal of Homosexuality, 42*(1), 29-51.

Minichiello, V., Mariño, R., Browne, J., & Jamieson, M. (2000). Commercial sex between men: A prospective diary-based study. *Journal of Sex Research, 37*, 151-160.

Minichiello, V., Mariño, R., Browne, J. & Jamieson, M. 1998. A review of male to male commercial sex encounters. *Venereology: The Interdisciplinary, International Journal of Sexual Health*, 11, 32-42.

Nourisis, M.J. (1998). *Statistical Package for the Social Sciences for Windows*. Version 9.0. Chicago, IL: SPSS.

Ratnapala, N. (1999). Male sex work in Sri Lanka. In P. Aggleton (Ed.), *Men who sell sex: International perspectives on male prostitution and HIV/AIDS* (pp. 213-222). Philadelphia, PA: Temple University Press.

Scott, J., Minichiello, V., Marino, R., Harvey, G.P., Jamieson, M., & Browne, J. (2004). Understanding the new context of the male sex work industry. *Journal of Interpersonal Violence*, 20, 263-269.

Sex Workers Outreach Project. (2003). Web: *http://www.swop.org.au*. Accessed January 2004.

Simon, P. M., Morse, E. V., Balson, P. M., Osofsky, H. J., & Gaumer, H. R. (1993). Barriers to human immunodeficiency virus related risk reduction among male street prostitutes. *Health Education Quarterly*, 20, 261-273.

Simon, P. M., Morse, E. V., Osofsky, H. J., Balson, P. M., & Gaumer, H. R (1992). Psychological characteristics of a sample of male street prostitutes. *Archives of Sexual Behavior, 21*, 33-44.

Snell, C. L. (1991). Help-seeking behavior among young street males. *Smith College Studies in Social Work, 61*, 293-305.

Weber, A. E., Craib, K. J., Chan, K., Martindale, S., Miller, M. L., Schechter, M. T., & Hogg, R. S. (2001). Sex trade involvement and rates of human immunodeficiency virus positivity among young gay and bisexual men. *International Journal of Epidemiology, 30*, 1449-1454.

Weinberg, M. S., Worth, H., & Williams, C. J. (2001). Men sex workers and other men who have sex with men: How do their HIV risks compare in New Zealand? *Archives of Sexual Behavior, 30*, 273-286.

West, D. J., & de Villiers, B. (1993). *Male prostitution*. New York, NY: Harrington Park Press, an imprint of The Haworth Press, Inc.

Ziersch, A., Gaffney, J., & Tomlinson, D. R. (2000). STI prevention and the male sex industry in London: Evaluating a pilot peer education programme. *Sexually Transmitted Infections, 76*(6), 447-453.

Exploring Commercial Sex Encounters in an Urban Community Sample of Gay and Bisexual Men: A Preliminary Report

Juline A. Koken, MA
Jeffrey T. Parsons, PhD
Joseph Severino, PhD(c)
David S. Bimbi, PhD(c)

SUMMARY. Prior research on gay and bisexual men who are paid for sex has been shaped by the bias towards sampling street-based men. Fewer studies have sampled men who pay for sex, and fewer still have

Juline A. Koken, Jeffrey T. Parsons, Joseph Severino, and David S. Bimbi are affiliated with the Center for HIV/AIDS Educational Studies and Training (CHEST). Juline A. Koken, Jeffrey T. Parsons, and David S. Bimbi are affiliated with the Graduate Center of the City University of New York. Jeffrey T. Parsons also has affiliations with Hunter College of the City University of New York.

Address correspondence to: Jeffrey T. Parsons, PhD, Professor, Department of Psychology, Hunter College of the City University of New York, 695 Park Avenue, New York, NY 10021 (E-mail: jeffrey.parsons@hunter.cuny.edu).

The Sex and Love Project was supported by the Hunter College Center for HIV/AIDS Educational Studies and Training (CHEST), under the direction of Dr. Parsons. The authors acknowledge the contributions of other members of the Sex and Love Project team–Whitney Missildine, Joseph C. Punzalan, Diane Tider, Jason Van Ora, Kalil Vicioso. They also thank David Frost and Elana Rosof for their assistance with the preparation of this manuscript.

[Haworth co-indexing entry note]: "Exploring Commercial Sex Encounters in an Urban Community Sample of Gay and Bisexual Men: A Preliminary Report." Koken, Juline A. et al. Co-published simultaneously in *Journal of Psychology & Human Sexuality* (The Haworth Press, Inc.) Vol. 17, No. 1/2, 2005, pp. 197-213; and: *Contemporary Research on Sex Work* (ed: Jeffrey T. Parsons) The Haworth Press, Inc., 2005, pp. 197-213. Single or multiple copies of this article are available for a fee from The Haworth Document Delivery Service [1-800-HAWORTH, 9:00 a.m. - 5:00 p.m. (EST). E-mail address: docdelivery@haworthpress.com].

attempted to identify men who report both paying and being paid for sex. The goal of this study was to obtain a descriptive "snapshot" of commercial sex encounters (CSEs) in a sexually active community sample of gay and bisexual men. Men completed a brief survey at a series of gay community events. Nearly half of the men reported paying for and/or having been paid for sex. Respondents who had been paid for sex were younger, more likely to be HIV positive, and reported more unsafe sex and substance use than non-CSE experienced men. Those who had paid or been paid for sex in the previous three months reported greater sexual risk behaviors than those who had not. These findings indicate that CSE experienced men remain a group at risk for infection or transmission of HIV and other STIs, as well as substance use or abuse. Implications for intervention are discussed. *[Article copies available for a fee from The Haworth Document Delivery Service: 1-800-HAWORTH. E-mail address: <docdelivery@haworthpress.com> Website: <http://www.HaworthPress.com> © 2005 by The Haworth Press, Inc. All rights reserved.]*

KEYWORDS. Male sex workers, gay/bisexual, clients, HIV, drug use

A review of the history of male sex work parallels in many ways the history of the psychological study of homosexuality (for a recent comprehensive review, see Minton, 2002). Moving from a literature that sought to "explain" these men and their clients from a perspective of deviancy or pathology (Caukins & Coombs, 1975; Sagarin, & Jolly, 1997), the advent of the AIDS epidemic shifted the focus on men who are paid for sex as "vectors of disease transmission" (Morse, Simon, Osofsky, Balson, & Gaumer, 1991; Vanwesenbeeck, 2001). While the study of homosexuality has moved away from the deviancy model (Minton, 2002), and towards a more non-judgmental effort at understanding men who have sex with men, the research literature on men who have sex with men for money is only recently beginning to follow suit (Browne & Minichiello, 1996; Minichiello et al., 1999; 2000; Koken, Bimbi, Parsons, & Halkitis, 2004; Parsons, Bimbi, & Halkitis, 2001; Parsons, Koken, & Bimbi, 2004; Vanwesenbeeck, 2001).

The majority of past research on men who are paid for sex to date has predominantly drawn from samples of street-based populations who are often adolescent, homeless, and engaging in "survival sex" (i.e., the exchange of sex for money, drugs or shelter) (Vanwesenbeeck, 2001). Alternatively, men have been drawn from psychiatrists' case histories

(Caukins & Coombs, 1975) with the a priori assumption of pathology, as illustrated in the title of one piece: "Prostitution: Profession and pathology" (Sagarin & Jolly, 1997). The findings of these studies have then too often been generalized to all men who are paid for sex, ignoring the diversity of experience across venues of sex work and individual differences.

The advent of the AIDS epidemic shifted much of the social scientific study of men who are paid for sex from a focus on deviancy to one of disease transmission. At first this literature scapegoated these men as responsible for the transmission of HIV into the heterosexual community (Gattari & Spizzichino, 1992; Morse et al., 1991); later, an extensive body of research showed that men who are paid for sex consistently use condoms during sexual encounters with their clients (Browne & Minichiello, 1996; Estcourt et al., 2000; Estep, Waldorf, & Marotta, 1992; Joffe & Dockrell, 1995; Minichiello et al., 2000; Overs, 1991; Parsons, Bimbi, & Halkitis, 2001; Parsons, Koken, & Bimbi, 2004; Perkins, Prestage, Sharp, & Lovejoy, 1994; Pleak & Meyer-Bahlburg, 1990; Ziersch, Gaffney, & Tomlinson, 2000). The role of men who pay for sex as potential sources of the transmission of HIV or other sexually transmitted infections (STIs) has largely been neglected, due perhaps in part to the difficulty in accessing this hidden population (Gomes do Espirito Santo & Etheridge, 2002). In fact, men who pay for sex have been understudied in the psychological literature, especially in the United States, where prostitution remains criminalized and clients a "hidden" population (Vanwesenbeeck, 2001).

In addition to problems of sampling, prior study of individuals who pay or are paid for sex has often been weakened by bias introduced via unexamined a priori assumptions about those who engage in commercial sex as workers or clients (Ditmore, 2002; Koken et al., 2004; Pheterson, 1990; Vanwesenbeeck, 2001). Such studies (Caukins & Coombs, 1975; Sagarin & Jolly, 1997; Morse et al., 1991) have contributed to the labeling and stigmatization of this already marginalized group (Koken et al., in press). However, recent research has begun to re-focus the picture of the commercial sex encounter away from a narrow, individual centered view to one that encompasses commercial sex encounters (CSEs) as events negotiated and enacted between two (or more) individuals within the larger sociocultural context (Browne & Minichiello, 1996; Knox, 1998; Minichiello et al., 1999; 2000). This trend in commercial sex research approaches men who pay or are paid for sex, risk factors, and interventions from a more holistic approach.

While street-based men have come to represent the image of the man who is paid for sex, men who work indoors have been largely neglected in the United States as a population of study. Indoor venues where men who are paid for sex work include bars, escort agencies and brothels; men may also work independently from home by advertising their services in gay newspapers or, more recently, via the World Wide Web. The use of the Internet as a point of contact between men who are paid for sex and the men who pay them seems to be increasing (Gaffney, 2003; Parsons et al., 2001; Parsons, Koken, & Bimbi, 2004). Recent coverage of this phenomenon in the gay media indicates that male escorting has become increasingly popular and less stigmatized in the gay community (Liberman, 2001). The lack of research on men who work indoors in the United States has resulted in a body of literature that has been biased towards men who work on the street, which is too often generalized to all men who are paid for sex. This begs the question of whether sampling bias has to some extent skewed past research findings (Van der Poel, 1992).

Several studies have indicated that men who work indoors differ substantially from street based men. Qualitative research with Internet-based MSWs has shown that the independence afforded by working indoors means that they can be more selective about their clients and the sexual activities they engage in, charge more for their services, and have greater control over their work schedule (Koken et al., 2004). Street based men are also at greater risk for arrest or victimization than men who work indoors (Calhoun & Weaver, 1996; Joffe & Dockrell, 1995).

In an effort to balance the majority of past research in the United States which has sampled mostly street-based men, and has scarcely sampled the men who pay them at all, the goal of this exploratory study was to approach CSEs from a community oriented perspective. The purpose of this study was to obtain a descriptive "snapshot" of how CSEs in the United States are enacted within the urban gay and bisexual community in terms of frequency, HIV and STI-related risk behaviors, and demographic characteristics.

METHOD

Participants and Procedure

Men ($n = 1072$) attending one of two large lesbian, gay, bisexual, and transgendered (LGBT) community events in New York City, completed a brief paper and pencil survey. Respondents who reported being sexually active in the previous three months outside of a monogamous relationship ($n = 660$) were selected for the purposes of this study. Individuals attending the event were approached and invited to complete a survey by a member of the research team. Individuals who agreed to respond were given a survey on a clipboard and a pencil, and were encouraged to move to a nearby seating area for privacy. The first page of the survey served as the assent form. The survey took approximately 10 to 15 minutes to complete. The response rate was high, with approximately 83.8% of individuals approached consenting to participate. A movie pass was given as an incentive for completing the survey.

Measures

Demographics. Characteristics were assessed using fill-in-the-blank measures of age, a race/ethnicity checklist, an HIV status checklist (positive, negative, don't know/untested, refuse to answer), and lifetime history of infection with an STI other than HIV ("have you ever had or been diagnosed with any of the following . . ." followed by a checklist of STIs), and a sexual orientation checklist (gay/lesbian/homosexual, bisexual, heterosexual, refuse to answer).

Sexual Behaviors. Respondents completed a series of questions pertaining to their sexual experiences. These questions assessed the respondent's sexual risk behaviors, such as having engaged in unprotected anal insertive or receptive intercourse. The response option to these questions offered agreement choices ranging from "never" to "1-2 times," "3-5 times," "6-9 times," "10 or more times," or "don't know." Experiences with CSEs were also measured with a yes or no question ("have you ever paid for sex?" Or "have you ever been paid for sex?"); those who responded yes were then asked "about how many times in the last year?" As these questions measured behavior, not identity, men who responded affirmatively will be referred to in this paper as "men who paid/were paid for sex" in order to avoid labeling respondents inappropriately as "sex workers" or "clients" when they may not have self-identified as such.

Substance Use. Substance use was measured with a yes or no response option for use "ever," "in the last three months," and "with sex." The substances were assessed individually and included crystal methamphetamine, ketamine, cocaine, crack, amyl nitrates ("poppers"), GHB, ecstasy, and marijuana. Additionally, a variable summing the number of substances used was created in order to measure overall levels of substance use by respondents.

Community Norms for CSEs. A series of questions intended to measure proximal (a phenomenon which may or may not occur in one's immediate social circle) versus distal (the broader social context) norms concerning the commonality of sex work in the gay/bisexual community were included (for example, "how common do you think it is for your friends to pay for sex? How common do you think it is for men in the gay community to get paid for sex?"). Response options to these questions ranged from "0" (not at all common) to "3" (very common).

Data Analysis

Only the data of single or non-monogamous men who reported sex in the previous three months were selected for analysis, resulting in a final sample of 660 men. This selection was performed as men who are not sexually active or sexually active only within a monogamous relationship are unlikely to be a major factor in HIV and STI transmission within the community. The majority of the subsample included in these analyses were White, HIV-negative, and had a mean age of 35.9 ($SD = 10$) (for a detailed breakdown of demographic characteristics, see Table 1). Two differences emerged between the sub-sample of 660 and the full sample of 1072 men: men in the sub-sample were significantly younger (F (1, 465) = 4.54, $p = .03$) and they were also more likely to self report being HIV positive (χ^2 (1) = 11.24, $p = .001$).

All analyses for this study were performed using SPSS to assess frequency data. Chi-Square, t-tests, and one-way ANOVAs were utilized to compare means and test for differences across groups. Respondents were grouped as follows: those reporting ever experiencing a CSE, by category (i.e., paid for sex, were paid for sex, or both), and a general group collapsing all those with CSE experience in the prior year to allow for comparison against those who never had such experience. Comparisons of drug use between the categories of CSE experienced men and those without CSE experience were performed by randomly selecting 100 of the non-experienced men. This balanced the cell sizes of CSE experienced men by category and those without such experience, allowing for a less skewed comparison. The sub-categories (paid for sex, were paid for sex, both) within the group which reported CSE experience in the last year were quite small, due in part to the amount of missing data on this item. For this reason all comparisons were performed

TABLE 1. Sample Characteristics

Race/Ethnicity	Frequency	Percent
African-American	57	8.6
Asian/Pacific Islander	56	8.5
European/White	426	64.5
Hispanic/Latino	79	12.0
Middle Eastern/Arab	6	0.9
Native American	11	1.7
Mixed	25	3.8
Sexual Identity		
Gay/homosexual	604	91.5
Bisexual	49	7.4
Heterosexual	6	0.9
Refuse to answer	1	0.2
Self-Reported Serostatus		
HIV-negative	419	63.5
HIV-positive	57	8.6
Untested/not reported	49	7.4
Relationship Status		
Single, not dating	217	32.9
Single, casually dating	272	41.2
Partnered, non-monogamous	159	24.1
Total	660	100.0

either with those who reported a lifetime history of CSE according to category, those who reported any CSE experience in the prior year, and those with no history of CSE experience.

RESULTS

Nearly half (42.7%, $n = 283$) of the men in the sample reported *ever* having had a CSE: of these men, 36.5% ($n = 103$) reported paying for sex, 36.9% ($n = 104$) had been paid for sex; while 26.6% ($n = 75$) reported having both been paid for sex as well as having paid for sex. No differences were found between men according to their category of CSE experience and their relationship status or sexual identity. Those who had been paid for sex were found to differ from others in several ways. Men who had been paid for sex were significantly younger ($M = 33.3$,

$SD = 9.31$) than men who reported paying for sex ($M = 40.5$, $SD = 9.23$) (F (3, 658) = 14.26, $p = .001$), and were significantly more likely to report unprotected anal receptive sex (χ^2 (3) = 18.50, $p < .000$) and unprotected anal insertive intercourse (χ^2 (3) = 15.22, $p = .002$) with their casual partners. Men who had been paid were also more likely to report being HIV-positive than those who paid for sex or those without CSE experience (χ^2 (6) = 16.67, $p = .011$).

Differences in drug use frequency were assessed across groups according to category of CSE experience (i.e., paid for sex, were paid, both, neither). Three one-way ANOVAs were performed to examine group differences for lifetime history of drug use, drug use within the last three months, and drug use with sex. Significant findings were followed by LSD post-hoc tests. On a combined measure of lifetime history of substance use (where the number of substances used was summed), men who had been paid for sex ($M = 4.69$, $SD = 2.57$) and those who reported paying and being paid ($M = 4.64$, $SD = 2.78$) reported higher levels of lifetime drug use than those reporting paying for sex ($M = 3.65$, SD = 2.31) and those reporting no CSEs ($M = 3.10$, $SD = 2.12$) (F (3, 561) = 16.48, $p = .000$). When examining the reported number of substances used within the last three months, men who had been paid for sex ($M = 2.56$, $SD = 2.26$) and those with experience in both sides of CSE transactions ($M = 2.29$, $SD = 2.47$) reported significantly more drug use than those without CSE experience ($M = 1.48$, $SD = 1.62$) and those who had paid for sex ($M = 1.18$, $SD = 1.26$) F (3, 558) = 9.67, $p = .001$. This finding was echoed by the rates of drug use when having sex: men who had been paid for sex ($M = 1.97$, $SD = 2.22$) and those reporting both paying and being paid for sex ($M = 1.79$, $SD = 2.15$) reported using more drugs with sex than men who paid for sex ($M = 1.18$, $SD = 1.26$) or those with no CSE experience ($M = 1.00$, $SD = 1.28$) (F (3,539) = 11.03, $p = .001$). For a complete breakdown of substance type and use by CSE category, see Table 2.

Upon examining respondents who reported current (within the previous year) sex work experience, the sub-sample reduces to only 75 gay and bisexual men (26.6% of the original 282 men who reported a lifetime history of CSE experience out of the total 660). Of these, 41 (54.7%) of these reported having been paid for sex, 19 (25.3%) had paid for sex, and 15 (20%) reported having engaged in both activities. A significant age difference was found across the groups (F (3, 138) = 6.39, $p < .000$). Post-hoc analysis (LSD) showed that men who paid for sex had a mean age of 41.95 ($SD = 10.06$), while those who reporting having been

TABLE 2. Prevalence (%) of Drug Use by Category of Sex Work Experience

Substance	History	Role in CSE experience				χ^2 (3)	p
		Were Paid (n = 90)	Paid for (n = 86)	Both (n = 63)	Neither (n = 89)		
Crystal	Ever	41.7	21.9	25	11.5	21.76	.000
	Last 3 mo	54.5	11.4	20.5	11.4	22.20	.000
	With sex[1]	55.3	13.2	23.7	7.9	22.33	.000
Cocaine	Ever	33.5	25.0	26.2	15.2	22.77	.000
	Last 3 mo	41.0	19.7	27.9	11.5	17.21	.001
	With sex	41.9	14.0	30.2	14.0	13.93	.003
Crack	Ever	23.3	18.6	48.8	9.3	27.35	.000
	Last 3 mo	n.a.	n.a.	n.a.	n.a.	n.a.	n.a.
	With sex	n.a.	n.a	n.a.	n.a.	n.a.	n.a.
Ecstasy	Ever	39.9	21.0	21.0	18.2	19.92	.000
	Last 3 mo	40.7	22.0	18.6	18.6	8.37	.039
	With sex	37.5	22.5	22.5	17.5	4.66	n.s.
GHB	Ever	45.8	15.3	28.8	10.2	21.33	.000
	Last 3 mo	n.a.	n.a.	n.a.	n.a.	n.a.	n.a.
	With sex	n.a.	n.a	n.a.	n.a.	n.a.	n.a.
Ketamine	Ever	40.6	21.9	24.0	13.5	16.71	.001
	Last 3 mo	38.7	25.8	22.6	12.9	4.99	n.s.
	With sex	n.a.	n.a.	n.a.	n.a.	n.a.	n.a.
Poppers	Ever	33.2	24.9	23.5	18.4	20.20	.000
	Last 3 mo	36.9	22.5	24.3	16.2	18.58	.000
	With sex	36.7	21.4	25.5	16.3	16.64	.001

[1]All 'with sex' frequencies reflect sex under the influence of a substance within the prior three months

paid for sex were approximately a decade younger (M = 31.49, SD = 8.25).

When taken as one group of those reporting a CSE in the past year (collapsing men who had paid and/or been paid for sex together, due to the small cell sizes) and compared with the men who reported not having had a CSE, the men with past year CSE experience were more likely to report any unprotected anal sex (χ^2 (1) = 7.28, p = .005) and having ever been infected with an STI other than HIV (χ^2 (1) = 9.95, p = .001). Further analysis shows that both unprotected anal insertive (χ^2 (1) = 4.203, p = .04) and anal receptive (χ^2 (1) = 4.28, p = .039) sex were significant. The number of sex partners men reported for the previous year may be contributing to this finding. Men with no CSE in the past year reported significantly fewer sexual partners (t = -3.46; p = .001), with a mean of 8.34 (SD = 13.3) partners in the last year, as compared to the CSE experienced group, which averaged 13.64 (SD = 22.1) partners in the last year.

On a set of questions designed to assess the proximal versus distal norms of CSEs, respondents indicated that they felt being paid or paying for sex was less common among their friends than it was in the general "gay community" (t = -23.52, p = .000; t = -28.78, p = .000).

DISCUSSION

Perhaps the most striking feature of this sample was that nearly half of the 660 respondents reported having paid or been paid for sex at some point in their life. While only a small percentage of respondents reported engaging in this behavior in the previous three months, it would appear that CSE transactions and the people involved with them are a relatively common, even integral, part of the sexual landscape in the urban gay and bisexual male community. While past research has often contributed to the labeling and marginalization of this population, and legal prohibition of sex work remains in every state of the United States (with limited exception in Nevada), previous qualitative research on the experience of stigma in the lives of male escorts indicates that sex work does not appear to be *as* heavily stigmatized within the gay community as it remains in the larger mainstream (heterosexual) culture (Koken et al., 2004). The findings of the present study lend weight to this perspective.

However, the response to the measure of community norms for sex work items (the questions designed to assess the proximal versus distal norms of CSEs), indicates that *some* measure of stigma does remain attached to CSEs. Men indicated that they felt being paid or paying for sex was less common among their friends than it was in the general "gay community." When considering the large number of respondents with

CSE experience alongside this finding, it is almost as if the message coming from the data reads "everyone's doing it, except for *my* friends." While there may still be a minimal amount of social opprobrium against the exchange of sex for money, these encounters were widely acknowledged as a feature of the community.

An unexpected feature of this sample was the finding of an overlap between those who paid or had been paid for sex. These men were behaviorally distinct from the discrete categories of men who paid for sex, those who were paid for it, or those without CSE involvement (see Table 2). Men who reported having both paid and been paid for sex seemed to fall between men who had engaged in only one or the other type of CSE on the continuum of risk behaviors such as unsafe sex or substance use. This phenomenon calls for future exploration; greater study is needed to determine the temporal ordering of these behaviors (i.e., were the men paid for sex first and paying for it later, or vice versa?) as well as the special characteristics of this population. There seems to be little previous literature on this "both" group, perhaps reflective of the common study methodology of approaching men who get paid or pay for sex as discrete groups.

Previous work with a sample of gay and bisexual male Internet escorts (Parsons et al., 2001; Parsons, Koken, & Bimbi, 2004; Koken et al., 2004) hinted at the blurring of the boundary between client and escort. Some of the men interviewed reported having hired escorts before becoming one; others engaged in "trade," a practice where two escorts would meet for sex without charging each other for the "session." The present study shows more definitively that men who pay or get paid for sex should be approached as part of a continuum of sexual practice, and future research in this area should allow for the possibility of this overlap in the data collection process.

Distressing differences between the categories of CSE involved or non-involved men were found in the present sample. It does appear that men who are paid for sex, and to a lesser extent those who pay them, remain a group especially at risk for infection by HIV and other STIs. As mentioned previously, those men who reported both paying and being paid for sex fell in between the two groups in terms of their risk behavior. Their vulnerability is further confirmed by the greater incidence of lifetime STI infection reported by CSE experienced men when compared to non-CSE experienced men. This trend echoes the results of a recent longitudinal study performed in Montreal, Canada (Roy et al., 2002), which uncovered similar trends in risk, as well as an overlap between paid and paid for sex. Unfortunately, this study did not separate men who both were paid and paid for sex from those who were solely paid for it, preventing direct comparison of our findings on this category of men with their sample.

The fact that the men in our study who reported having been paid for sex were more likely to report unprotected anal sex with their casual partners than men who were not sex work experienced indicates a continued need for health behavior interventions among this population. This need is especially urgent given the greater rate of HIV infection among men who were paid for sex in this sample than among those who were not. However, a more detailed assessment of the sexual practices of men who are paid for sex, including an examination of risk behavior by serostatus of partner, is necessary to ascertain whether the increased sex risk behaviors noted in this study resulted from calculated risk (i.e., a harm reduction approach such as "serosorting"), an impulsive "slip," or perhaps as a result of coercion.

Also of concern were the higher levels of substance use reported by CSE involved men. Those who reported having been paid for sex or both being paid as well as paying for sex reported a greater lifetime history of substance use than men who paid for sex or those without CSE experience; where verifiable (some cells became too small for statistical comparison), this was again found for drug use in the prior three months and with sex (see Table 2). While the data did not allow for sophisticated analysis of any possible relationship between sex transactions and substance use, the higher rate of substance use among men who were paid for sex and men with both types of CSE experience indicates that men who are paid for sex have specific health needs that clearly should be addressed with health behavior interventions and continued community education on the risks of substance use and abuse. The fact that several studies (Colfax et al., 2001; Halkitis, Parsons, & Wilton, 2003; Klitzman, Pope, & Hudson, 2000; Lee, Galanter, Dermatis, & McDowell, 2003) have found a link between risky sex and "club drug" (e.g., crystal methamphetamine, ketamine, cocaine, ecstasy, and GHB) use among gay and bisexual men makes this phenomenon an even greater public health concern.

Before the finding of greater substance use and risky sex among men with CSE experience may be placed into a meaningful framework, further research on the contexts of substance use and risky sex among this population is needed to understand the directionality of this relationship. In some recent studies (Kalichman, Weinhardt, DiFonzo, & Austin, 2002; Kalichman, Cain, Zweben, & Swain, 2003), sensation seeking was associated with alcohol use and risky sexual behavior among some gay and bisexual men. It is possible that substance use may have a similar relationship among gay and bisexual men as well, although the present data cannot directly affirm this. Qualitative research methods may be better suited to eliciting a more nuanced picture of the sociocultural meanings and contexts attached to CSEs among urban gay and bisexual men, as well as the risk factors that may impact CSE involved men.

Some factors should be taken into consideration when evaluating the results of this study. The LGBT events where this data were collected required paid admission, which may limit the generalizability of these findings to gay and bisexual men with some degree of disposable income. However, as the majority of research to date on commercial sex encounters has sampled street-based men who are paid for sex, and rarely men who pay for sex, the sampling of a more diverse and financially comfortable population may provide a balance to data collected previously, especially in the United States. Additionally, as the venues of data collection were marketed towards the LGBT community, they were less likely to attract non-gay identified men who have sex with men, and as such, these findings should not be generalized to this population.

Another limitation of the data concerns the measurement of sexual risk behaviors used for the present study, which unfortunately did not distinguish between casual partners accompanied by a financial exchange and those that were for unpaid pleasure alone. The measure also failed to distinguish between sexual risk with HIV seroconcordant versus serodiscordant partners. This prevents assessment of "serosorting" among respondents. Serosorting is a harm reduction approach involving unprotected sex with men of the same HIV serostatus, used by some gay men to reduce the risk of transmitting HIV.

Past research has shown that while male sex workers usually practice safer sex with clients, they may be less likely to do so with their non-paid partners (for a review see Vanwesenbeeck, 2001). While the current study did not assess for this, it is recommended that future research in this area do so. Following the findings of the prior research cited above, it is advisable that interventions and programming targeted at men who pay or are paid for sex take into account the different types of sex partners CSE experienced men have in order to maximize their effectiveness. Additionally, our data did not allow for statistical comparison of risk behaviors between men who are *currently* engaged in commercial sex practices by category (i.e., respondents who were paid or paid for sex in the previous three months) and those who are not CSE experienced, due to limitations imposed by the imbalance in cell sizes.

Finally, while past research on men who are paid for sex (Browne et al., 1996; Parsons, Bimbi, & Halkitis, 2001) has shown that the venue of work (i.e., street, escort agency, Internet, etc.) impacts upon the nature of risk encountered by these men, our study did not assess for this. While it is most likely that the majority of the men who reported being paid for sex were not street based, due to the presence of an admission fee to gain entry to the community events where the surveys were administered, this cannot be determined due to limitations in the measurement of our data. For these reasons, the findings presented here should be taken as descriptive and exploratory in nature.

Future research in this area would do well to continue to explore commercial sex transactions between men as a phenomenon based in the sociocultural location within which CSEs occur. Studies that sample sex work involved men as part of the larger gay and bisexual community should assess the cultural meanings attached to these interactions in order to gain a better understanding of how commercial sex is practiced and perceived by members of the community. Qualitative research methods would be well suited to this endeavor.

While this study sampled mostly gay and bisexually identified men who paid and/or were paid for sex, few studies in the United States to date have explored such men who may be heterosexually identified (but not street-based) and thus unlikely to be reached through research on the gay and bisexual community. These men are likely to differ in their expectations, desires and practices during CSEs; this would be an excellent area for future study.

It is reassuring that CSE involved men may be reached by health behavior interventions aimed at the general sexually active gay community (as indicated by the ease with which this group was accessed through community events targeting the LGBT community at large). Community based organizations attempting to reach this population may benefit by taking a two pronged approach: first by continuing efforts to reduce risky sexual behavior among sexually active gay and bisexual men, especially young men; and second, by designing specific interventions that address the special needs of CSE involved men. The use of multiple efforts at intervention and education may have the best chance at reaching a greater number of sexually active men who pay and/or are paid for sex.

Prior research on the perceived needs of male escorts indicates that this group would benefit from interventions that extend beyond the simple mandate "use a condom every time" (Parsons et al., 2001). Qualitative data obtained from in depth interviews with male escorts who advertise on the Internet, a rapidly growing sector of men who are paid for sex (Gaffney, 2003; Koken et al., 2004), indicate that these men desire health promotion programs that would educate them about a variety of life management issues, such as how to file taxes, invest their earnings, negotiate the legal restrictions on their work, and interact with clients. Interventions that incorporate this information as part of an effort to aid men who are paid for sex in maintaining safer sex practices not only with their clients, but also with casual partners, may be more successful at recruiting these men than designs that solely emphasize the practice of safer sex.

Organizations that serve male escorts, such as the online program "HOOKonline.com" have noted these needs and are engaged in addressing them. Community based organizations and service providers would do well to reach out and learn from existing sex work advocates and educators, as well as recent excellent research in this area (such as Ditmore, 2002; Ziersch et al., 2000) in order to design programming that is respectful, sensitive to the needs of men who pay or are paid for sex, and presented in an accessible and appealing format.

The findings of this study underscore the need for further research on male sex work as a phenomenon based within the larger urban gay and bisexual male community. The advantages of collecting data from a large sample of men attending a GLBT community event are many. First, the great majority of research on male sex work has too often been limited to street based samples of men who are paid for sex; the present study thus provides data on a larger, more diverse population of sex work involved men. Second, the information gathered in this study on the characteristics of gay and bisexually identified men who pay for sex also provides insight on this rarely sampled group. Commercial sex encounters are an integral part of the urban gay and bisexual landscape, and the findings presented here suggest that continued research on the contextual aspects of CSEs is warranted.

REFERENCES

Browne, J., & Minichiello, V. (1996). The social and work context of commercial sex between men: A Research note. *The Australian and New England Journal of Sociology, 32*, 86-92.

Caukins, S., & Coombs, N. (1975). The Psychodynamics of male prostitution. *American Journal of Psychotherapy, 30*, 441-452.

Colfax, G.N., Mansergh, G., Guzman, R., Vittinghoff, E., Marks, G., Rader, M., et al. (2001). Drug use and sexual risk behavior among gay and bisexual men who attend circuit parties: A Venue-based comparison. *Journal of Acquired Immune Deficiency Syndrome, 28,* 373-379.

Coutinho, R.A., van Andel, R.L.M., & Rijsdijk, T.J. (1988). Role of male prostitutes in the spread of sexually transmitted diseases and human immuno-deficiency virus. *Genitourinary Medicine, 64,* 207-208.

Ditmore, M. (2002). Reaching out to sex workers. In *Reaching the hardly reached.* Program for Appropriate Technology and Health, Network of Sex Work Projects.

Estcourt, C.S., Marks, C., Rohrsheim, R., Johnson, A.M., Donovan, B., & Mindel, A. (2000). HIV, sexually transmitted infections, and risk behaviors in male commercial sex workers in Sydney. *Sexually Transmitted Infections, 76,* 294-298.

Estep, R., Waldorf, D., & Marotta, T. (1992). Sexual behavior of male prostitutes. In J. Huber, & B. E. Schneider (Eds.), *The Social context of AIDS.* Newbury Park, CA: Sage Publications.

Gaffney, J. (2003, June). *Working together with male sex workers (MSW) in London.* Paper presented at the European Network of Male Prostitution, Hamburg, Germany.

Gattari, P., & Spizzichino, L. (1992). Behavioral patterns and HIV infection among drug using transvestites practicing prostitution in Rome. *AIDS Care, 4,* 83-88.

Gomes do Espirito Santo, M.E., & Etheredge, G.D. (2002). How to reach clients of female sex workers: A Survey "by surprise" in brothels in Dakar, Senegal. *Bulletin of the World Health Organization, 80,* 709-713.

Halkitis, P.N., Parsons, J.T., & Wilton, L. (2003). An Exploratory study of contextual and situational factors related to methamphetamine use among gay and bisexual men in New York City. *Journal of Drug Issues, 33,* 413-432.

Joffe, H., & Dockrell, J.E. (1995). Safer sex: Lessons from the male sex industry. *Journal of Community & Applied Social Psychology, 5,* 333-346.

Kalichman, S. C., Cain, D., Zweben, A., & Swain, G. (2003). Sensation seeking, alcohol use and sexual risk behaviors among men receiving services at a clinic for sexually transmitted infections. *Journal of Studies on Alcohol. 64,* 564-9.

Kalichman, S. C., Weinhardt, L., DiFonzo, K., Austin, J., & Luke, W. (2002). Sensation seeking and alcohol use as markers of sexual transmission risk behavior in HIV-positive men. *Annals of Behavioral Medicine, 24,* 229-35.

Klitzman, R.L., Pope, H.G., Jr., & Hudson, J.I. (2000). MDMA ("Ecstasy") abuse and high-risk sexual behaviors among 169 gay and bisexual men. *American Journal of Psychiatry, 157,* 1162-1164.

Koken, J.A., Bimbi, D.S., Parsons, J.T., & Halkitis, P.N. (2004). The Experience of stigma among gay and bisexual male Internet escorts. *Journal of Psychology &Human Sexuality, 16*(1), *13-32.*

Knox, M.P. (1998). Negotiations and relationships among male sex workers and clients in Liverpool, Merseyside, United Kingdom. In Elias, J. E. (Ed.), *Prostitution: On whores, hustlers, and johns* (pp. 236-259). Amherst, NY: Prometheus.

Lee, S.J., Galanter, M., Dermatis, H., & McDowell, D. (2003). Circuit parties and patterns of drug use in a subset of gay men. *Journal of Addictive Diseases, 22,* 47-60.

Liberman, V. (2001). Show me the money: Instinct's guide to hiring and becoming an escort. *Instinct*, 6, 36-40.

Morse, E.V., Simon, P.M., Osofsky, H.J., Balson, P.M., & Gaumer, H.R. (1991). The Male street prostitute: A Vector for transmission of HIV infection into the heterosexual world. *Social Science and Medicine*, 32, 535-539.

Minichiello, V., Marino, R., Browne, J., Jamieson, M., Peterson, K., Reuter, B., et al. (1999). A Profile of the clients of male sex workers in three Australian cities. *Australian and New Zealand Journal of Public Health*, 23, 511-418.

Minichiello, V., Marino, R., Browne, J., Jamieson, M., Peterson, K., Reuter, B., et al. (2000). Commercial sex between men: A Prospective diary-based study. *The Journal of Sex Research*, 37, 151-160.

Minton, H. (2002). *Departing from deviance: A History of homosexual rights and emancipatory science in America*. Chicago, IL: The University of Chicago Press.

Overs, C. (1991). *To work or not to work? Questions facing HIV-positive sex workers*. National AIDS Bulletin (Australia).

Parsons, J.T., Bimbi, D.S., & Halkitis, P.N. (2001). Sexual compulsivity among gay/bisexual male escorts who advertise on the internet. *Journal of Sexual Addiction and Compulsivity*, 8, 113-123.

Parsons, J.T., Koken, J.A., & Bimbi, D.S. (2004). The Use of the Internet by gay and bisexual male escorts: Sex workers as sex educators. *AIDS Care*, 16(8), 1021-1035.

Perkins, R. (1985). Motivations. In: *Being a prostitute: Prostitute women and prostitute men* (pp. 213-222). Sydney, Australia: George Allen Sunwin.

Perkins, R., Prestage, G., Sharp, R., & Lovejoy, F. (1994). *Sex work and sex workers in Australia*. Sydney, Australia: University of New South Wales Press, Ltd.

Pheterson, G. (1990). The category "prostitute" in scientific inquiry. *Social Science and Medicine*, 32, 535-539.

Pleak, R.R., & Meyer-Bahlburg, H.F.L. (1990). Sexual behavior and AIDS knowledge of young male prostitutes in Manhattan. *Journal of Sex Research*, 27, 557-588.

Roy, J.L., Otis, J., Vincelette, J., Alary, M., Zunzunegui, M. V., Gaudreault, M., et al. (2002, July). *Characteristics of Omega study participants who have received money or drugs in exchange for sex*. Poster presented at the XIV International AIDS Conference, Barcelona, Spain.

Sagarin, E., & Jolly, R.J. (1997). Prostitution: Profession and pathology. In: Schlesinger, L.B., & Revitch, E.R. (Eds.), *Sexual dynamics of anti-social behavior* (pp. 9-30, 2nd ed.). Springfield, IL: Charles C. Thomas, Publisher.

Salamon, E. (1989). The homosexual escort agency: Deviance disavowal. *The British Journal of Sociology*, 40, 1-21.

Vanwesenbeeck, I., (2001). Another decade of social scientific work on sex work: A Review of research 1990-2000. *Annual Review of Sex Research*, 12, 242-300.

Ziersch, A., Gaffney, J., & Tomlinson, D.R. (2000). STI prevention and the male sex industry in London: Evaluating a pilot peer education program. *Sexually Transmitted Infections*, 76, 447-453.

Index

Page numbers followed by the letter "t" designate tables; page numbers in *italics* designate figures. *See also* cross-references designate detailed lists of subtopics.

BOOK ORDER FORM!

Order a copy of this book with this form or online at:
http://www.HaworthPress.com/store/product.asp?sku=5630

Contemporary Research on Sex Work

_____ in softbound at $24.95 ISBN-13: 978-0-7890-2964-5 / ISBN-10: 0-7890-2964-2.
_____ in hardbound at $49.95 ISBN-13: 978-0-7890-2963-8 / ISBN-10: 0-7890-2963-4.

COST OF BOOKS _____

POSTAGE & HANDLING _____
US: $4.00 for first book & $1.50
for each additional book
Outside US: $5.00 for first book
& $2.00 for each additional book.

SUBTOTAL _____

In Canada: add 7% GST. _____

STATE TAX _____
CA, IL, IN, MN, NJ, NY, OH, PA & SD residents
please add appropriate local sales tax.

FINAL TOTAL _____

If paying in Canadian funds, convert
using the current exchange rate,
UNESCO coupons welcome.

❑ BILL ME LATER:
Bill-me option is good on US/Canada/
Mexico orders only; not good to jobbers,
wholesalers, or subscription agencies.

❑ Signature _____

❑ Payment Enclosed: $_____

❑ PLEASE CHARGE TO MY CREDIT CARD:
❑ Visa ❑ MasterCard ❑ AmEx ❑ Discover
❑ Diner's Club ❑ Eurocard ❑ JCB

Account #_____

Exp Date _____

Signature _____
(Prices in US dollars and subject to change without notice.)

PLEASE PRINT ALL INFORMATION OR ATTACH YOUR BUSINESS CARD

Name

Address

City   State/Province   Zip/Postal Code

Country

Tel   Fax

E-Mail

May we use your e-mail address for confirmations and other types of information? ❑ Yes ❑ No We appreciate receiving
your e-mail address. Haworth would like to e-mail special discount offers to you, as a preferred customer.
We will never share, rent, or exchange your e-mail address. We regard such actions as an invasion of your privacy.

Order from your **local bookstore** or directly from
The Haworth Press, Inc. 10 Alice Street, Binghamton, New York 13904-1580 • USA
Call our toll-free number (1-800-429-6784) / Outside US/Canada: (607) 722-5857
Fax: 1-800-895-0582 / Outside US/Canada: (607) 771-0012
E-mail your order to us: orders@HaworthPress.com

For orders outside US and Canada, you may wish to order through your local
sales representative, distributor, or bookseller.
For information, see http://HaworthPress.com/distributors

(Discounts are available for individual orders in US and Canada only, not booksellers/distributors.)

The Haworth Press Inc.

Please photocopy this form for your personal use.
www.HaworthPress.com

BOF05

Oct. 26/07

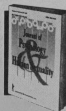